keep the beat™
recipes

deliciously healthy family meals

D1737581

U.S. Department of Health and Human Services
National Institutes of Health

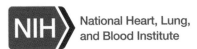
National Heart, Lung, and Blood Institute

NIH Publication No. 10-7531
December 2010
Reprinted January 2013

™ Keep the Beat is a trademark of the U.S. Department of Health and Human Services (HHS).
® *We Can! Ways to Enhance Children's Activity & Nutrition, We Can!*, and the *We Can!* logos are registered trademarks of HHS.

contents

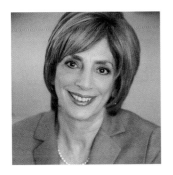

from the NHLBI director

Dear Friends:

With everyone's busy schedules, how can you find time each day for the whole family to be together? Try spending family time in the kitchen, preparing healthy meals, and teaching your children to build lifelong healthy eating habits.

The National Heart, Lung, and Blood Institute (NHLBI) is pleased to present this new Keep the Beat™ cookbook to help busy parents who want to make meal preparation a family affair. *Keep the Beat™ Recipes: Deliciously Healthy Family Meals* features delicious, heart healthy recipes, just like NHLBI's *Keep the Beat™ Recipes: Deliciously Healthy Dinners*. The cookbook showcases new dishes that were created especially for the NHLBI by a Culinary Institute of America-trained chef/instructor and father of two. We even tested the recipes with parents and school-aged children to make sure they liked them.

The cookbook also provides tips for involving children in meal preparation. The appendix is loaded with information on meal planning, cooking, and nutrition for families and children.

Keep the Beat™ Recipes: Deliciously Healthy Family Meals was developed in partnership with the NIH's *We Can!*® (**W**ays to **E**nhance **C**hildren's **A**ctivity & **N**utrition) program—a national education program to help children stay at a healthy weight. For more information on both Keep the Beat™ healthy eating and *We Can!*, see "Hungry for More?" (Resources) on the inside back cover.

I hope you enjoy preparing and eating these meals with your family!

Best wishes,

Susan B. Shurin, M.D.
Acting Director
National Heart, Lung, and Blood Institute

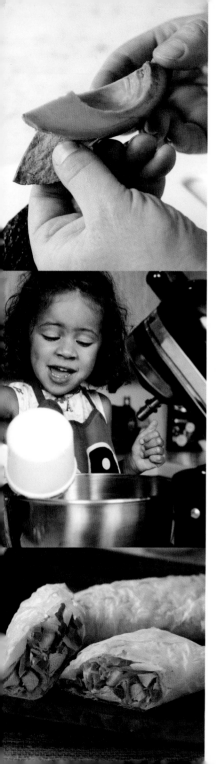

acknowledgments

The National Heart, Lung, and Blood Institute (NHLBI) would like to give special thanks to those involved with the development of *Keep the Beat™ Recipes: Deliciously Healthy Family Meals.*

Recipes were developed by David Kamen, PC^{III}/C.E.C., C.C.E., C.H.E., Chef/Instructor at the Culinary Institute of America.

Recipe testing was conducted by Northern Illinois University (NIU) Nutrition and Dietetics and Program students and faculty and managed by Beverly Henry, Ph.D., R.D., Associate Professor. Recipes were sampled by school children at NIU Child Development Laboratory, Paul T. Wright Elementary School, and Malta Elementary School.

Food photographs were taken by Ben Fink Photography.

The NHLBI staff who provided technical expertise and direction for the cookbook include Karen Donato, S.M., Janet de Jesus, M.S., R.D., Melinda Kelley, Ph.D., and Melissa McGowan, M.H.S., CHES.

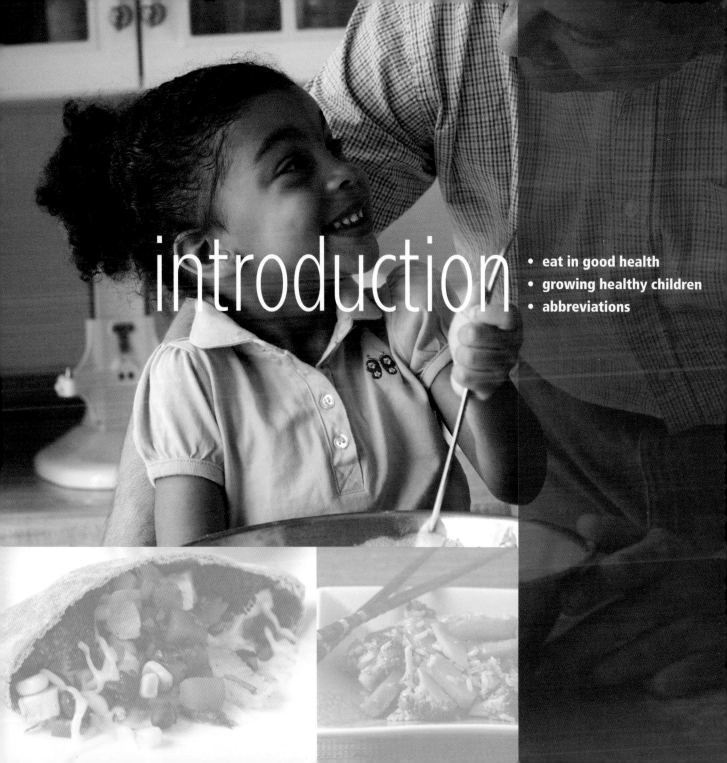

introduction

- eat in good health
- growing healthy children
- abbreviations

introduction

Do you feel challenged to serve your family healthy meals each day? Nutritious food doesn't have to be bland or take a long time to prepare. You can prepare healthy recipes that taste great—and that your children will love. *Keep the Beat*™ *Recipes: Deliciously Healthy Family Meals* dishes up all that and more. With kid-tested recipes, such as Southwestern Beef Roll-Ups, Hawaiian Huli Huli Chicken, and Mexican Lasagna, these meals are sure to be winners on your table.

Keep the Beat™ *Recipes: Deliciously Healthy Family Meals* contains more than 40 recipes that are quick, simple, and taste great. The recipes were created for the National Heart, Lung, and Blood Institute (NHLBI) by a Culinary Institute of America-trained chef/instructor and father of two. The cookbook features:

- Deliciously healthy entrees, side dishes, and snacks that appeal to both children and adults

- Recipes that are budget friendly, multicultural, and relatively quick and easy for busy families to make

- Symbols that help identify types of recipes, such as "leftover friendly"

- Tips to show children how to prepare recipes with the help of parents and caregivers

eat in good health

Eating healthfully and being physically active are two ways to help lower your risk and your children's risk of heart disease and other conditions. And it has been shown that eating and physical activity habits are formed early in life.

One way to eat a healthy diet is to choose a variety of foods. Variety matters, because no food has all of the nutrients that your heart and the rest of your body need. A healthy eating plan is one that:

- Emphasizes fruits, vegetables, whole grains, and fat-free and low-fat milk and milk products

- Includes lean meat, poultry, fish, beans, eggs, and nuts

- Is low in saturated fat, *trans* fat, cholesterol, sodium, and added sugars

Also, think about what your family drinks. Choose water, fat-free or low-fat milk, and low- or no-calorie beverages as a substitute for regular, sweetened beverages. If you have a family member who is lactose intolerant, lactose-free fat-free and low-fat milk are good options.

The recipes in this cookbook were created to fit into your family's healthy eating plan. They use lean cuts of meat, poultry without the skin, fish, beans, whole grains, fruits, vegetables, and small amounts of vegetable oil—plus lots of herbs and spices for flavor. Most of all, these recipes offer a delicious way for your family to eat together.

growing healthy children

Keep the Beat™ Recipes: Deliciously Healthy Family Meals was developed jointly with the National Institutes of Health (NIH) *We Can!*® program. *We Can!* (Ways to Enhance Children's Activity & Nutrition) is a national education program designed to give parents, caregivers, and entire communities a way to help children stay at a healthy weight. The NIH and the NHLBI recognize that children's adoption of healthy food habits at a young age can help them maintain a healthy weight throughout life.

As parents, you can do a lot to help your children learn healthy eating habits and help them maintain a healthy weight. Research shows that introducing fruits, vegetables, whole grains, and other healthier foods in the early years increases the chance that children will like these foods. Involving children in cooking and meal preparation can motivate them to try new, healthy foods—and is a good way to spend time together as a family. The following tips can help you encourage and support your children's healthier food habits:

- Set a good example.
- Go food shopping together, and ask your children to choose healthier foods they want to try.
- Offer a variety of foods, particularly "GO foods" (foods lowest in calories and fat, and most "nutrient dense"; for more information, see page 91).
- Encourage children to try new foods from each food group.
- Offer the same foods to everyone in the family (don't be a "short order cook").
- Help your children learn to recognize when they've had enough.

- Make mealtime family time.

- Make healthier food fun to help your child be excited to eat it.

- Provide fruits and vegetables for snacks.

For more information on each of these tips and other food and nutrition information for children, see "Hungry for More?" (Resources) on the inside back cover.

The appendixes in this cookbook also feature helpful resources on healthy cooking for busy families, including:

- Time-saving tips for busy families

- Guidance on how much children should eat daily

- Hints on getting your children involved in the kitchen

- Common cooking measurements and equivalents

- Frequently asked questions

Enjoy a Keep the Beat™ recipe with your family today, and eat in good health!

abbreviations

Recipes use the following abbreviations:

C .... cup

lb .... pound

oz .... ounce

pkg .... package

pt .... pint

qt .... quart

Tbsp .... tablespoon

tsp .... teaspoon

Nutrient lists use the following abbreviations:

g .... gram

mg .... milligram

guide to recipe symbols

Healthier Classics
Classic favorites that are made healthier by reducing fat, calories, and/or sodium. Healthier classics also could have more vegetables or whole grains added than original versions.

Leftover Friendly
Recipes that use leftover ingredients to help save cooking time.

Chefs in Training
Tips for getting children involved in meal preparation.

Healthy Eating Two Ways
Simple tips to serve a recipe two ways to please picky eaters and other family members.

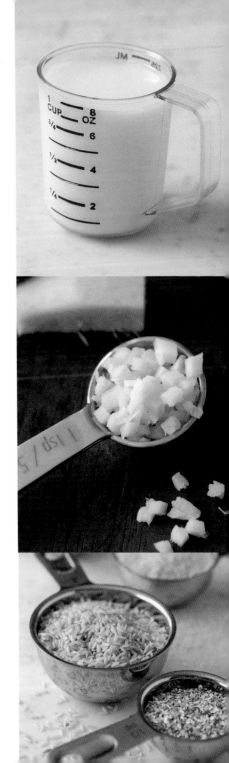

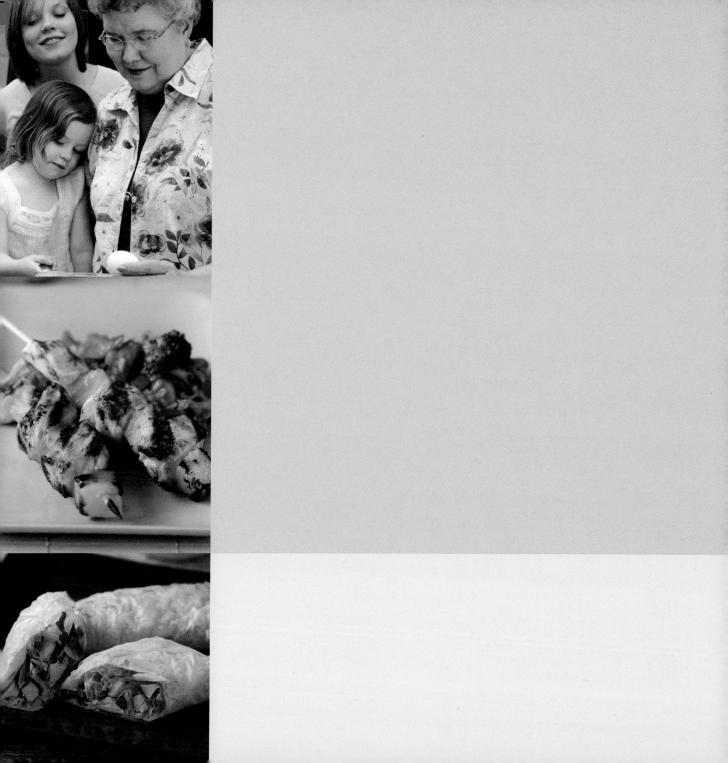

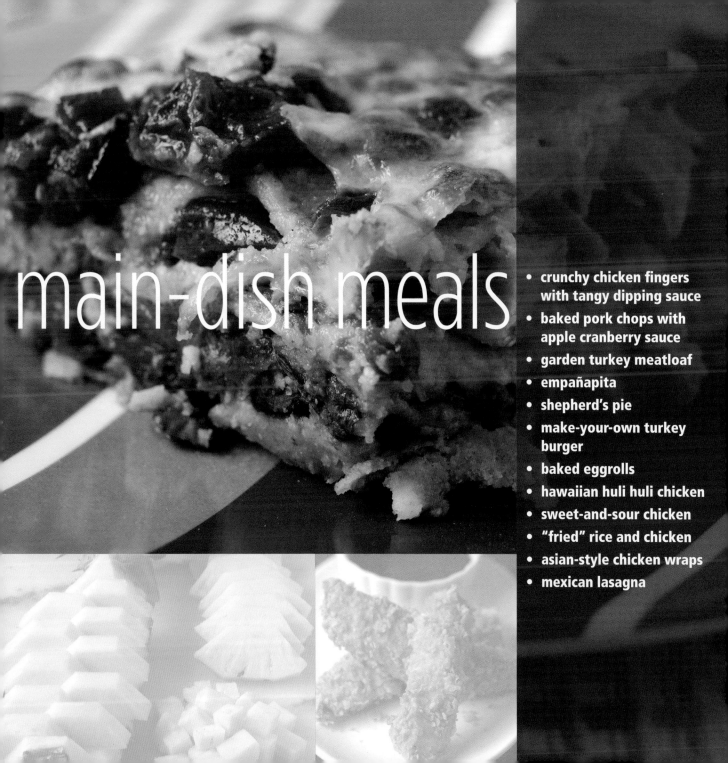

main-dish meals

- crunchy chicken fingers with tangy dipping sauce
- baked pork chops with apple cranberry sauce
- garden turkey meatloaf
- empañapita
- shepherd's pie
- make-your-own turkey burger
- baked eggrolls
- hawaiian huli huli chicken
- sweet-and-sour chicken
- "fried" rice and chicken
- asian-style chicken wraps
- mexican lasagna

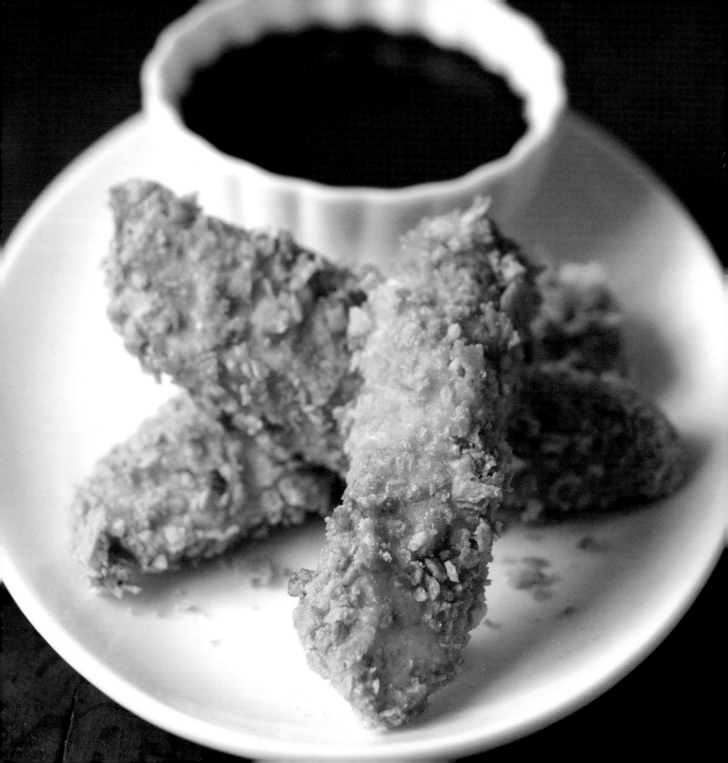

crunchy chicken fingers with tangy dipping sauce

try this family classic, made healthier with baked chicken and a yummy dipping sauce

For chicken:

½ tsp	reduced-sodium crab seasoning (or substitute ¼ tsp paprika and ¼ tsp garlic powder for a sodium-free alternative)
¼ tsp	ground black pepper
1 Tbsp	whole-wheat flour
12 oz	boneless, skinless, chicken breast, cut into 12 strips
2 Tbsp	fat-free (skim) milk
1	egg white (or substitute 2 Tbsp egg white substitute)
3 C	cornflake cereal, crushed

For sauce:

¼ C	ketchup
¼ C	100 percent orange juice
¼ C	balsamic vinegar
2 Tbsp	honey
2 tsp	deli mustard
1 tsp	Worcestershire sauce

1. Preheat oven to 400 °F.
2. Mix crab seasoning, pepper, and flour in a bowl.
3. Add chicken strips, and toss well to coat evenly.
4. Combine milk and egg white in a separate bowl, and mix well. Pour over seasoned chicken, and toss well.
5. Place crushed cornflakes in a separate bowl. Dip each chicken strip into the cornflakes, and coat well. Place strips on a nonstick baking sheet. (Discard any leftover cornflake mixture.)
6. Bake chicken strips for 10–12 minutes (to a minimum internal temperature of 165 °F).
7. Meanwhile, prepare the sauce by combining all ingredients and mixing well.
8. Serve three chicken strips with ¼ cup dipping sauce.

Younger children can crush the cornflakes. Older children can dredge the chicken through the coating and mix the tangy sauce.

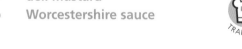 **prep time:** 10 minutes	**yield:** 4 servings	**each serving provides:**	
cook time: 12 minutes	**serving size:** 3 chicken strips, ¼ C sauce	calories	248

each serving provides:			
calories	248	carbohydrates	36 g
total fat	2 g	potassium	303 mg
saturated fat	1 g	vitamin A	4%
cholesterol	47 mg	vitamin C	16%
sodium	422 mg	calcium	6%
total fiber	1 g	iron	4%
protein	20 g		

Percent Daily Values are based on a 2,000 calorie diet.

baked pork chops with apple cranberry sauce

a wonderful fruit sauce adds the perfect touch to these pork chops—try serving
with a side of brown rice and steamed broccoli

For pork chops:

4	boneless pork chops (about 3 oz each)
¼ tsp	ground black pepper
1	medium orange, rinsed, for ¼ tsp zest *(use a grater to take a thin layer of skin off the orange; save the orange for garnish)*
½ Tbsp	olive oil

For sauce:

¼ C	low-sodium chicken broth
1	medium apple, peeled and grated (about 1 C) *(use a grater to make thin layers of apple)*
½	cinnamon stick (or ⅛ tsp ground cinnamon)
1	bay leaf
½ C	dried cranberries *(or substitute raisins)*
½ C	100 percent orange juice

1. Preheat oven to 350 °F.
2. Season pork chops with pepper and orange zest.
3. In a large sauté pan, heat olive oil over medium heat. Add pork chops, and cook until browned on one side, about 2 minutes. Turn over and brown the second side, an additional 2 minutes. Remove pork chops from the pan, place them on a nonstick baking sheet, and put in the oven to cook for an additional 10 minutes (to a minimum internal temperature of 160 °F).
4. Add chicken broth to the sauté pan and stir to loosen the flavorful brown bits. Set aside for later.
5. Meanwhile, place grated apples, cinnamon stick, and bay leaf in a small saucepan. Cook over medium heat until the apples begin to soften.
6. Add cranberries, orange juice, and saved broth with flavorful brown bits. Bring to a boil, and then lower to a gentle simmer. Simmer for up to 10 minutes, or until the cranberries are plump and the apples are tender. Remove the cinnamon stick.
7. Peel the orange used for the zest, and cut it into eight sections for garnish.
8. Serve one pork chop with ¼ cup of sauce and two orange segments.

If your children would prefer it without the sauce on top, serve a plain pork chop with separate sides of unsweetened applesauce, dried cranberries, and orange segments.

♥ prep time:	yield:	each serving provides:			
10 minutes	4 servings	calories	232	carbohydrates	25 g
		total fat	7 g	potassium	384 mg
cook time:	serving size:	saturated fat	2 g	vitamin A	2%
30 minutes	1 pork chop, ¼ C sauce,	cholesterol	50 mg	vitamin C	60%
	2 orange segments	sodium	42 mg	calcium	4%
		total fiber	2 g	iron	6%
		protein	18 g		

Percent Daily Values are based on a 2,000 calorie diet.

garden turkey meatloaf

this classic family favorite is made healthier with lean ground turkey
and colorful garden vegetables

For meatloaf:

2 C	assorted vegetables, chopped—such as mushrooms, zucchini, red bell peppers, or spinach *(Leftover Friendly)*
12 oz	99 percent lean ground turkey
½ C	whole-wheat breadcrumbs *(or substitute regular breadcrumbs)*
¼ C	fat-free evaporated milk*
¼ tsp	ground black pepper
2 Tbsp	ketchup
1 Tbsp	fresh chives, rinsed, dried, and chopped (or 1 tsp dried)
1 Tbsp	fresh parsley, rinsed, dried, and chopped (or 1 tsp dried)

Nonstick cooking spray

For glaze:

1 Tbsp	ketchup
1 Tbsp	honey
1 Tbsp	Dijon mustard

1. Preheat oven to 350 °F.
2. Steam or lightly sauté the assortment of vegetables.
3. Combine vegetables and the rest of the meatloaf ingredients in a large bowl. Mix well. Spray a loaf pan with cooking spray, and spread meatloaf mixture evenly in the pan.
4. Combine all ingredients for glaze. Brush glaze on top of the meatloaf.
5. Bake meatloaf in the oven for 45–50 minutes (to a minimum internal temperature of 165 °F).
6. Let stand for 5 minutes before cutting into eight even slices.
7. Serve two slices on each plate.

Tip: For picky eaters, try chopping vegetables in a food processer to make them smaller (and "hidden").

* Evaporated milk can be kept tightly sealed in the refrigerator for up to 3 days. Search the Keep the Beat™: Deliciously Healthy Eating Web site (http://hin.nhlbi.nih.gov/healthyeating) for other recipes using evaporated milk.

If you don't have leftover cooked vegetables, see basic cooking instructions in appendix D (page 103).

prep time:
10 minutes

cook time:
50–55 minutes

yield:
4 servings

serving size:
2 slices meatloaf

each serving provides:

calories	180	carbohydrates	17 g
total fat	2 g	potassium	406 mg
saturated fat	0 g	vitamin A	50%
cholesterol	34 mg	vitamin C	15%
sodium	368 mg	calcium	10%
total fiber	2 g	iron	15%
protein	25 g		

Percent Daily Values are based on a 2,000 calorie diet.

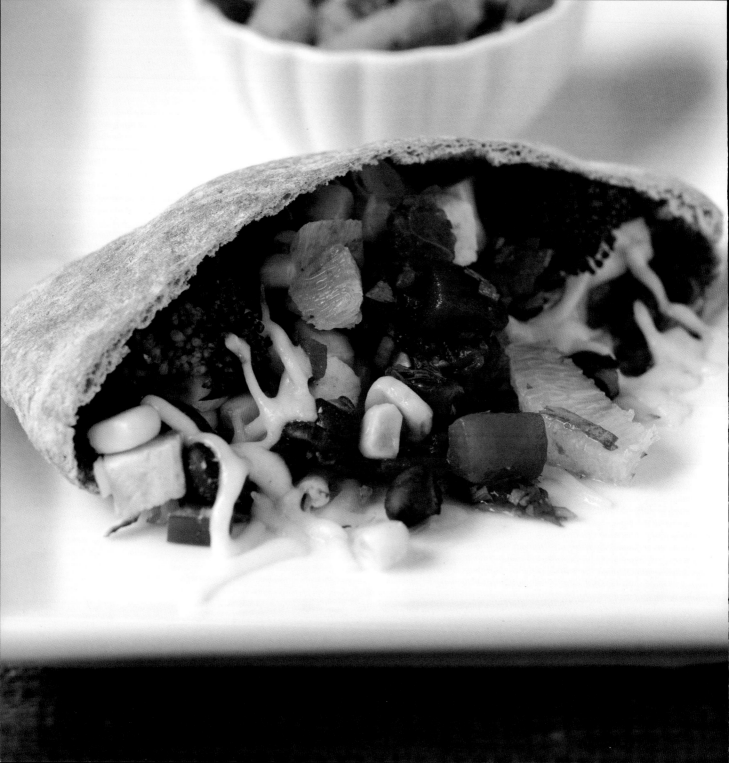

empañapita

similar to a Spanish empañada, this empaña"pita" uses pita bread for the shell

2   (6½-inch) whole-wheat pitas

1 C   **Tangy Salsa** *(see recipe on page 51)*

For filling:

2 C   **canned low-sodium black beans, rinsed**

2 C   **frozen broccoli, corn, and pepper vegetable mix, thawed** *(Leftover Friendly)*

2 C   **grilled boneless, skinless chicken breast, diced (about 4 small breasts)**

½ C   **shredded low-moisture part-skim mozzarella cheese**

1 Tbsp   **fresh cilantro, rinsed, dried, and chopped** *(or substitute 1 tsp dried coriander)*

2 Tbsp   **scallions (green onions), rinsed and chopped** *(or substitute red onions)*

1. Preheat oven to 400 °F.
2. Combine beans, vegetables, chicken, cheese, and seasonings. Mix well.
3. Cut pitas in half, and open the pockets. Divide filling evenly between the four halves (about 1½ cups each).
4. Place pitas on a nonstick baking sheet, and bake for about 10 minutes until the filling is hot, cheese melts, and chicken is reheated.
5. Serve each empañapita with ¼ cup of **Tangy Salsa**.

Note: If you can't find beans labeled "low sodium," compare the Nutrition Facts panels to find the beans with the lowest amount of sodium. Rinsing can help reduce sodium levels further.

If you don't have leftover cooked vegetables, see basic cooking instructions in appendix D (page 103).

Children can help stuff ingredients into the pita pockets.

		each serving provides:		
prep time: 10 minutes (20 minutes with homemade salsa)	**yield:** 4 servings	calories	373	carbohydrates 60 g
		total fat	4 g	potassium 741 mg
		saturated fat	1 g	vitamin A 180%
cook time: 10 minutes	**serving size:** 1 stuffed pita half, ¼ C Tangy Salsa	cholesterol	34 mg	vitamin C 50%
		sodium	374 mg	calcium 8%
		total fiber	14 g	iron 25%
		protein	27 g	

Percent Daily Values are based on a 2,000 calorie diet.

shepherd's pie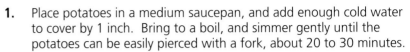

leftover chicken and vegetables make this classic dish quick and easy to prepare

For potatoes:

1 lb	Russet potatoes (or other white baking potatoes), rinsed, peeled, and cubed into ½-inch to ¾-inch pieces
¼ C	low-fat plain yogurt (or low-fat sour cream)
1 C	fat-free milk, hot
¼ tsp	salt
¼ tsp	ground black pepper
1 Tbsp	fresh chives, rinsed, dried, and chopped (or 1 tsp dried)

For filling:

4 C	mixed cooked vegetables—such as carrots, celery, onions, bell peppers, mushrooms, or peas (or a 1-lb bag frozen mixed vegetables) *(Leftover Friendly)*
2 C	low-sodium chicken broth
1 C	quick-cooking oats
1 C	grilled or roasted chicken breast, diced (about 2 small breasts) *(Leftover Friendly)*
1 Tbsp	fresh parsley, rinsed, dried, and chopped (or 1 tsp dried)
¼ tsp	ground black pepper
Nonstick cooking spray	

1. Place potatoes in a medium saucepan, and add enough cold water to cover by 1 inch. Bring to a boil, and simmer gently until the potatoes can be easily pierced with a fork, about 20 to 30 minutes.

2. While the potatoes are cooking, begin to prepare the filling. Combine the vegetables, chicken broth, and oats in a medium saucepan. Bring to a boil, and simmer gently until the oatmeal is cooked, about 5–7 minutes. Add chicken, and continue to simmer until heated through. Season with parsley and pepper. Hold warm until potatoes are ready.

3. When potatoes have about 5 minutes left to cook, preheat the oven to 450 °F.

4. When the potatoes are done, drain and dry them well, then mash with a potato masher or big fork.

5. Immediately add the yogurt, hot milk, and salt to the potatoes. Stir well until smooth. Season with pepper and chives.

6. Lightly spray an 8- by 8-inch square baking dish, or four individual 4-inch ceramic bowls, with cooking spray. Place filling in the bottom of prepared dish (about 2 cups each for individual bowls). Carefully spread potato mixture on top of the chicken and vegetables (about 1 cup each for individual bowls) so they remain in two separate layers.

7. Bake in the preheated oven for about 10 minutes, or until the potatoes are browned and chicken is reheated (to a minimum internal temperature of 165 °F). Serve immediately.

 If you don't have leftover cooked vegetables or chicken, see basic cooking instructions in appendix D (page 103).

prep time: 40 minutes	**yield:** 4 servings	**each serving provides:**
cook time: 10 minutes	**serving size:** ¼ of the baking dish or 1 individual bowl (about 1 C potatoes and 2 C chicken and vegetables)	

each serving provides:

calories	336	carbohydrates	54 g
total fat	4 g	potassium	957 mg
saturated fat	1 g	vitamin A	160%
cholesterol	31 mg	vitamin C	40%
sodium	302 mg	calcium	15%
total fiber	7 g	iron	15%
protein	24 g		

Percent Daily Values are based on a 2,000 calorie diet.

make-your-own turkey burger

let family members help prepare the meal by choosing their own burger ingredients

12 oz	99 percent lean ground turkey
2 Tbsp	fresh parsley, rinsed, dried, and chopped (or 2 tsp dried)
4	whole-wheat hamburger buns

Nonstick cooking spray

Burger ingredients:

1 C	fresh tomatoes, rinsed and diced (or canned no-salt-added diced tomatoes)
1 C	red onions, diced
1 C	white mushrooms, rinsed and sliced
1 C	part-skim shredded mozzarella cheese

1. Preheat oven to 350 °F.
2. Arrange burger ingredients (tomatoes, red onions, mushrooms, and mozzarella cheese) in separate bowls.
3. Ask each person to select ¼ cup total of his or her choice of ingredients. *(You may have leftover ingredients after this step—keep or freeze for use in other recipes!)*
4. Divide ground turkey into four parts on a plate.
5. Ask each person to combine his or her ¼ cup of burger ingredients with one portion of ground turkey and mix well to form a patty ½-inch to ¾-inch thick.
6. Brown burgers on a nonstick pan coated with cooking spray for 2–3 minutes on each side. Then, transfer burgers to a baking sheet coated with cooking spray and place in the preheated oven for about 10 minutes (to a minimum internal temperature of 165 °F).
7. Assemble burgers on buns, and serve.

 Each "chef" can help set out the ingredients and make his or her own burger.

prep time: 10 minutes	**yield:** 4 servings
cook time: 30 minutes	**serving size:** 1 burger with ¼ C mixed ingredients on a bun

each serving provides:

calories	308	carbohydrates	30 g
total fat	8 g	potassium	432 mg
saturated fat	3 g	vitamin A	15%
cholesterol	52 mg	vitamin C	20%
sodium	230 mg	calcium	4%
total fiber	4 g	iron	15%
protein	33 g		

Note: Nutritional information may vary depending on selection of ingredients.

Percent Daily Values are based on a 2,000 calorie diet.

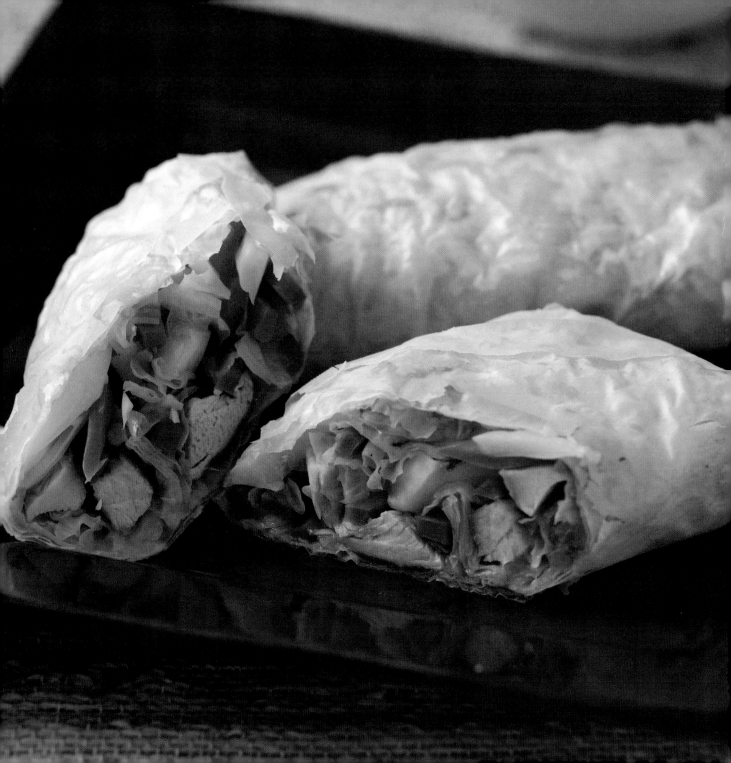

baked eggrolls

phyllo dough makes these eggrolls easy to roll—try with a side of **Wiki (Fast) Rice** (on page 61)

1 Tbsp	vegetable oil
2 tsp	sesame oil (optional)
2 tsp	ginger, minced (or ½ tsp dried)
2 tsp	garlic, minced (about 2 cloves)
4 C	cabbage (napa or Chinese), rinsed and shredded
2 C	carrots, peeled and sliced thinly on an angle (julienned)
2 C	grilled boneless, skinless chicken breast, cut into strips (about 4 small breasts) *(Leftover Friendly)*
1 tsp	lite soy sauce
8	phyllo dough sheets
Nonstick cooking spray	

1. Preheat oven to 400 °F.
2. Heat vegetable and sesame oils in a large wok or sauté pan over medium heat.
3. Add ginger and garlic. Stir fry quickly, about 30–45 seconds.
4. Add cabbage and carrots. Continue stir frying until the cabbage is soft, about 2–3 minutes.
5. Add chicken and soy sauce. Toss well and heat through.
6. Remove mixture from the pan, and place in a large colander to drain.
7. To assemble eggrolls, cover layers of phyllo with a damp cloth to stay moist. Place one sheet of phyllo dough on a cutting board. Spray it lightly with cooking spray. Top with another layer of phyllo dough, and spray again. Repeat for a total of four layers. Prepare a second stack with the remaining four layers.
8. Cut layered dough into four squares. Divide filling evenly (about 1 cup portions) into the center of each stack of squares. Fold one corner of the square into the middle (on top of the filling). Fold in the two sides, and roll the eggroll over so the folded parts are on the bottom.
9. Place the rolls on a nonstick baking sheet, and bake for 15–20 minutes, or until brown and crisp and chicken is reheated. Serve immediately.

Note: For guidance (with photos) on how to fold an eggroll, see the FAQs in appendix D (on page 104).

If you don't have leftover cooked chicken, see basic cooking instructions in appendix D (page 103).

prep time:	yield:	each serving provides:			
15–20 minutes	4 servings	calories	324	carbohydrates	30 g
		total fat	11 g	potassium	416 mg
cook time:	serving size:	saturated fat	2 g	vitamin A	230%
20 minutes	2 eggrolls	cholesterol	60 mg	vitamin C	45%
		sodium	320 mg	calcium	10%
		total fiber	3 g	iron	15%
		protein	26 g		

Percent Daily Values are based on a 2,000 calorie diet.

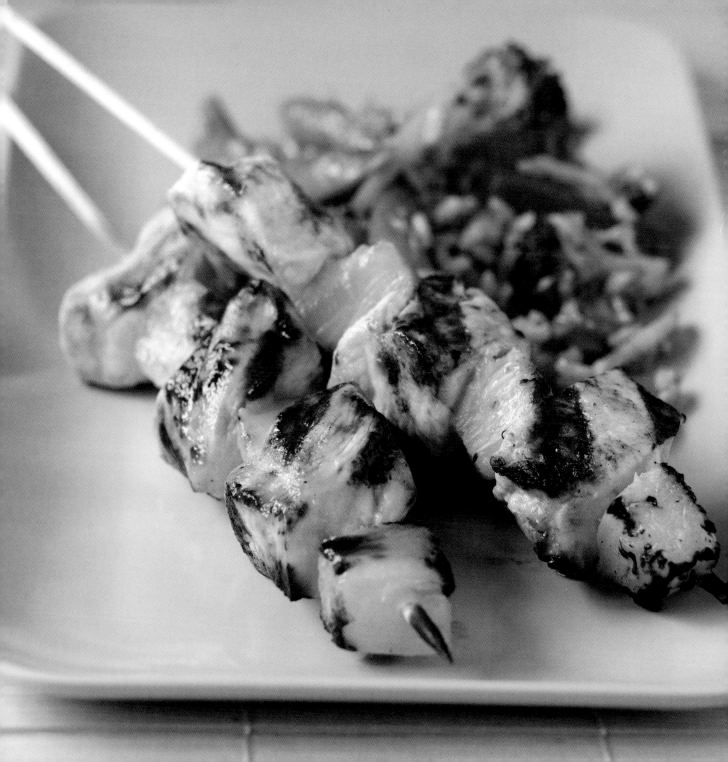

hawaiian huli huli chicken

so fun to eat that your children won't know it's healthy too—try serving with **Wow-y Maui Pasta Salad** (on page 57)

12 oz	boneless, skinless chicken breast, cut into 1-inch cubes (24 cubes) (about 2 large breasts)
1 C	fresh pineapple, diced (24 pieces) (or canned pineapple chunks in juice)
8	6-inch wooden skewers

For sauce:

2 Tbsp	ketchup
2 Tbsp	lite soy sauce
2 Tbsp	honey
2 tsp	orange juice
1 tsp	garlic, minced (about 1 clove)
1 tsp	ginger, minced

1. Preheat a broiler or grill on medium-high heat.
2. Thread three chicken cubes and three pineapple chunks alternately on each skewer.
3. Combine ingredients for sauce and mix well; separate into two bowls and set one aside for later.
4. Grill skewers for 3–5 minutes on each side. Brush or spoon sauce (from the bowl that wasn't set aside) onto chicken and pineapple about every other minute. Discard the sauce when done with this step.
5. To prevent chicken from drying out, finish cooking skewers in a 350 °F oven immediately after grilling (to a minimum internal temperature of 165 °F). Using a clean brush or spoon, coat with sauce from the set-aside bowl before serving.

Tip: Use leftover chicken and sauce leftover from step 5 of the **"Fried" Rice and Chicken** (on page 15).

Note: Skewers have sharp edges, so monitor younger children while eating, or take the chicken off the skewers for them.

Children can help mix the sauce and thread the chicken and pineapple on the skewers.

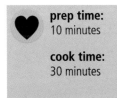

prep time:	yield:	each serving provides:			
10 minutes	4 servings	calories	156	carbohydrates	16 g
		total fat	2 g	potassium	255 mg
cook time:	serving size:	saturated fat	1 g	vitamin A	2%
30 minutes	2 skewers	cholesterol	47 mg	vitamin C	15%
		sodium	320 mg	calcium	2%
		total fiber	0 g	iron	6%
		protein	18 g		

Percent Daily Values are based on a 2,000 calorie diet.

sweet-and-sour chicken

sweet and sour flavors make a winning combination in this healthier version of a popular Chinese dish

1 bag	(12 oz) frozen vegetable stir-fry
1 Tbsp	peanut oil or vegetable oil
1 Tbsp	ginger, minced
1 Tbsp	garlic, minced (about 2–3 cloves)
1 Tbsp	scallions (green onions), rinsed and minced
2 Tbsp	rice vinegar
1 Tbsp	Asian hot chili sauce *(Healthy Eating Two Ways)*
2 Tbsp	brown sugar
1 Tbsp	cornstarch
1 C	low-sodium chicken broth
12 oz	boneless, skinless chicken breast, cut into thin strips
1 Tbsp	lite soy sauce

1. Thaw frozen vegetables in the microwave (or place entire bag in a bowl of hot water for about 10 minutes). Set aside until step 6.
2. Heat oil in a large wok or sauté pan over medium heat. Add ginger, garlic, and scallions, and stir fry until cooked, but not browned, about 2–3 minutes.
3. Add the rice vinegar, chili sauce, and brown sugar to the pan, and bring to a simmer.
4. In a bowl, mix cornstarch with chicken broth, and add to the pan. Bring to a boil over high heat, stirring constantly. Lower heat to a gentle simmer.
5. Add chicken, and stir continually for 5–8 minutes.
6. Add vegetables, and mix gently. Simmer with lid on to reheat, about 2 minutes.
7. Add soy sauce, and mix gently.
8. Divide into four even portions, and serve.

Tip: Try serving with a side of steamed rice.

Chili sauce may be too spicy for children—consider adding this ingredient individually at the table.

prep time: 15 minutes	**yield:** 4 servings		
cook time: 15 minutes	**serving size:** 3 oz chicken, 1 C vegetables		

each serving provides:

calories	221	carbohydrates	21 g
total fat	6 g	potassium	460 mg
saturated fat	1 g	vitamin A	90%
cholesterol	51 mg	vitamin C	45%
sodium	287 mg	calcium	6%
total fiber	3 g	iron	6%
protein	23 g		

Percent Daily Values are based on a 2,000 calorie diet.

"fried" rice and chicken

use leftovers from the **Hawaiian Huli Huli Chicken** (on page 13) to make this quick and easy weeknight meal

1	Tbsp	vegetable oil
1	tsp	garlic, minced (about 2 cloves)
1	C	no-salt-added diced tomatoes, with juice drained
4	C	assorted vegetables (or a 1-lb bag frozen mixed vegetables) *(Leftover Friendly)*
2	C	cooked brown rice *(Leftover Friendly)*
1	C	cooked boneless, skinless chicken breast, diced *(Leftover Friendly)*
¼	C	sauce from **Hawaiian Huli Huli Chicken** *(see recipe on page 13)*
1	Tbsp	lite soy sauce
½	Tbsp	sesame oil

1. Heat oil in a large wok or sauté pan.
2. Add garlic, and cook over medium heat until soft, but not browned, about 1 minute.
3. Add tomatoes, and continue to cook until they become slightly dry, about 5 minutes.
4. Add vegetables, and cook until heated through, about 3–5 minutes.
5. Add rice and chicken. Toss well, and cook until heated through, about 5–7 minutes.
6. Add soy sauce and sesame oil. Toss to incorporate, and serve.

Note: Substitute cooking spray for vegetable oil and save calories and fat.

This recipe is best prepared with leftover cold rice. If you don't have leftover cooked vegetables or chicken, see basic cooking instructions in appendix D (page 103).

prep time: 10 minutes	yield: 4 servings	**each serving provides:**			
		calories	407	carbohydrates	66 g
cook time: 20 minutes	serving size: 2 C rice and chicken	total fat	8 g	potassium	679 mg
		saturated fat	1 g	vitamin A	360%
		cholesterol	30 mg	vitamin C	15%
		sodium	394 mg	calcium	10%
		total fiber	11 g	iron	20%
		protein	22 g		

Percent Daily Values are based on a 2,000 calorie diet.

asian-style chicken wraps

delicious finger food that's just as healthy as it is fun to eat

For sauce:

1	small Jalapeno chili pepper, rinsed and split lengthwise—remove seeds and white membrane, and mince (about 1 Tbsp); for less spice, use green bell pepper
1 Tbsp	garlic, minced (about 2–3 cloves)
3 Tbsp	brown sugar or honey
½ C	water
½ Tbsp	fish sauce
2 Tbsp	lime juice (or about 2 limes)

For chicken:

1 Tbsp	peanut oil or vegetable oil
1 Tbsp	ginger, minced
1 Tbsp	garlic, minced (about 2–3 cloves)
12 oz	boneless, skinless chicken breast, cut into thin strips
1 Tbsp	lite soy sauce
1 Tbsp	sesame oil (optional)
1 Tbsp	sesame seeds (optional)

For wrap:

1	(small) head red leaf lettuce, rinsed, dried, and separated into single leaves large enough to create wrap
8	fresh basil leaves, whole, rinsed and dried
2 C	bok choy or Asian cabbage, rinsed and shredded

1. To prepare the sauce, add all ingredients to a saucepan, and bring to a boil over high heat. Remove from heat, and let sit in hot saucepan for 3–5 minutes. Chill in refrigerator for about 15 minutes, or until cold.

2. Prepare the chicken by heating oil in a large wok or sauté pan. Add ginger and garlic, and stir fry briefly until cooked, but not browned, about 30 seconds to 1 minute.

continued on page 17

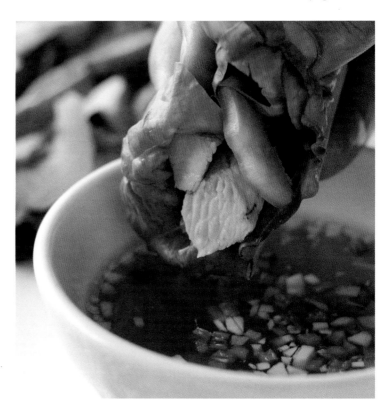

asian-style chicken wraps (continued)

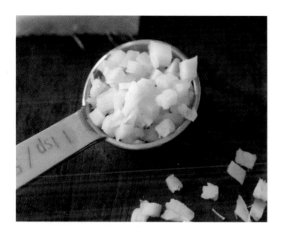

3. Add chicken, and continue to stir fry for 5–8 minutes.
4. Add soy sauce, sesame oil (optional), and sesame seeds (optional), and return to a boil. Remove from the heat, and cover with lid to hold warm in hot sauté pan.
5. Assemble each wrap: Place one red lettuce leaf on a plate, then add ½ cup chicken stir-fry, 1 basil leaf, and ¼ cup shredded cabbage and fold together. Serve two wraps with ¼ cup sauce.

CHEFS IN TRAINING

Children can help fill the wraps and mix the sauce.

prep time:	yield:	each serving provides:			
15 minutes	4 servings	calories	242	carbohydrates	17 g
		total fat	10 g	potassium	636 mg
cook time:	serving size:	saturated fat	2 g	vitamin A	170%
20 minutes	2 wraps, ¼ C sauce	cholesterol	47 mg	vitamin C	80%
		sodium	393 mg	calcium	20%
		total fiber	3 g	iron	15%
		protein	21 g		

Percent Daily Values are based on a 2,000 calorie diet.

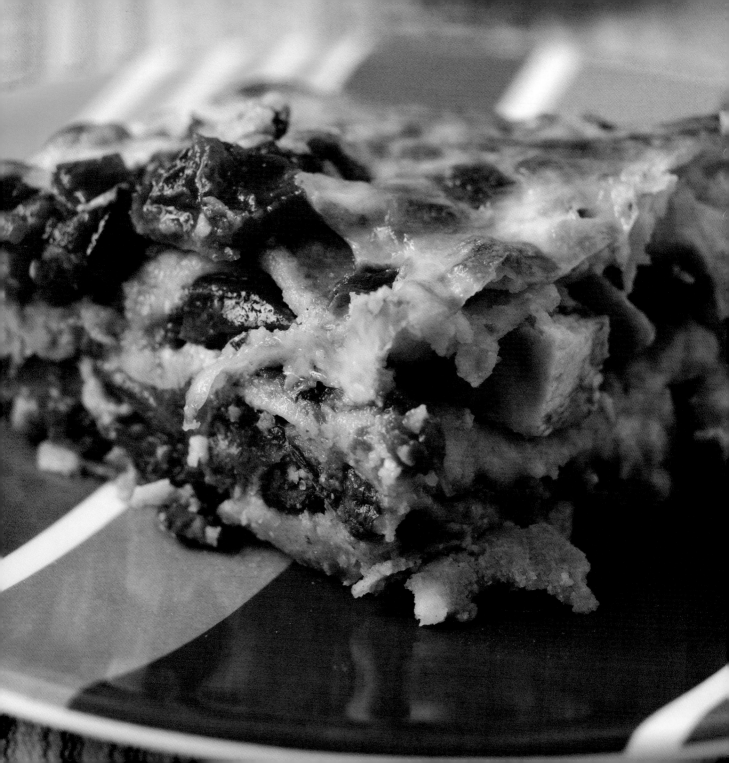

mexican lasagna

this festive twist on lasagna—and a quick weeknight meal—will make your family cheer "olé!"

10	6-inch corn tortillas
2 C	canned low-sodium black beans, rinsed
4 C	**Super Quick Chunky Tomato Sauce** *(see recipe on page 54) (Leftover Friendly)*
1½ C	Monterey Jack cheese, grated
1 bag	(10 oz) baby spinach leaves, rinsed
2 C	grilled chicken, diced *(Leftover Friendly)*
2 Tbsp	fresh cilantro, rinsed, dried, and chopped *(or substitute 1 tsp dried coriander)*

Nonstick cooking spray

1. Preheat oven to 400 °F.
2. Lightly spray a 9- by 13-inch baking pan with cooking spray. Place two to three corn tortillas on the bottom, trimming as necessary for a good fit.
3. Add beans, 1 cup tomato sauce, and ½ cup grated cheese. Top with two to three more corn tortillas.
4. Add 1 cup tomato sauce, spinach, and ½ cup cheese. Top with two more corn tortillas.
5. Add chicken and 1 cup tomato sauce. Top with two more corn tortillas.
6. Add 1 cup tomato sauce, ½ cup cheese, and cilantro.
7. Bake for 30 minutes, or until the cheese is melted and browned and chicken is reheated.
8. Let stand for 5 minutes. Cut into eight even squares, and serve.

Note: If you can't find beans labeled "low sodium," compare the Nutrition Facts panels to find the beans with the lowest amount of sodium. Rinsing can help reduce sodium levels further.

Children can help layer the "lasagna" ingredients.

If you don't have leftover cooked chicken, see basic cooking instructions in appendix D (page 103).

prep time:
10 minutes
(15 minutes with homemade sauce)

cook time:
35 minutes
(50 minutes with homemade sauce)

yield:
8 servings

serving size:
1 square

each serving provides:

calories	304	carbohydrates	31 g
total fat	10 g	potassium	550 mg
saturated fat	4 g	vitamin A	80%
cholesterol	52 mg	vitamin C	15%
sodium	275 mg	calcium	30%
total fiber	6 g	iron	15%
protein	23 g		

Percent Daily Values are based on a 2,000 calorie diet.

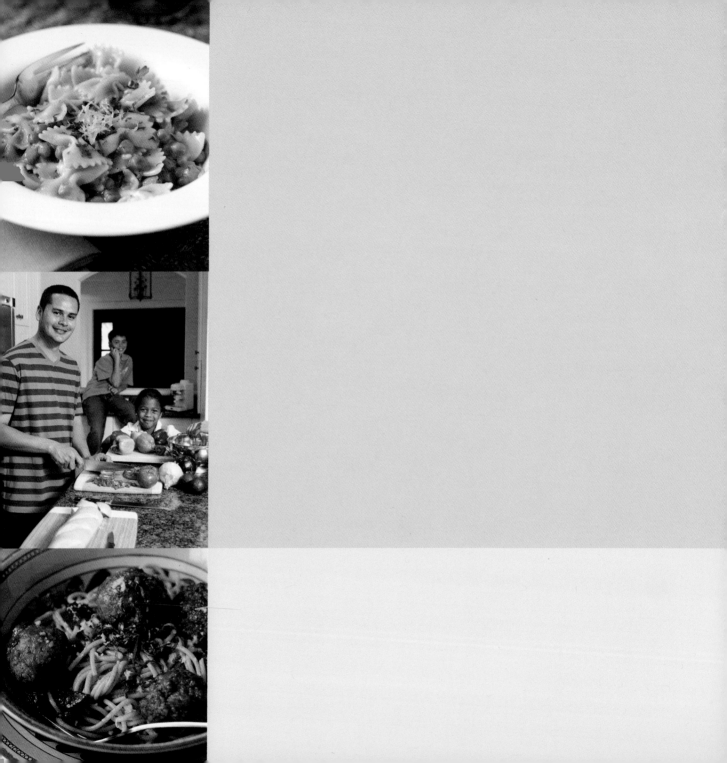

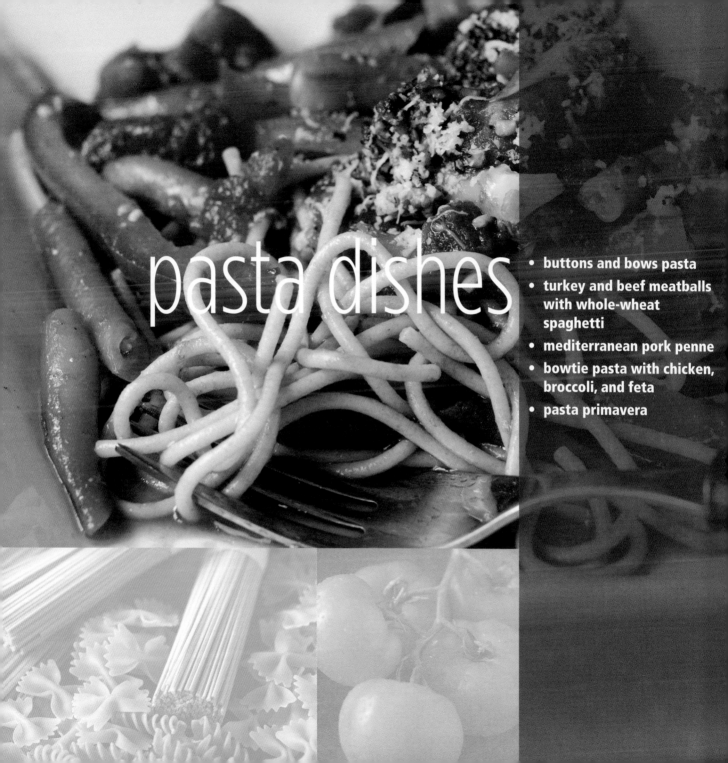

pasta dishes

- **buttons and bows pasta**
- **turkey and beef meatballs with whole-wheat spaghetti**
- **mediterranean pork penne**
- **bowtie pasta with chicken, broccoli, and feta**
- **pasta primavera**

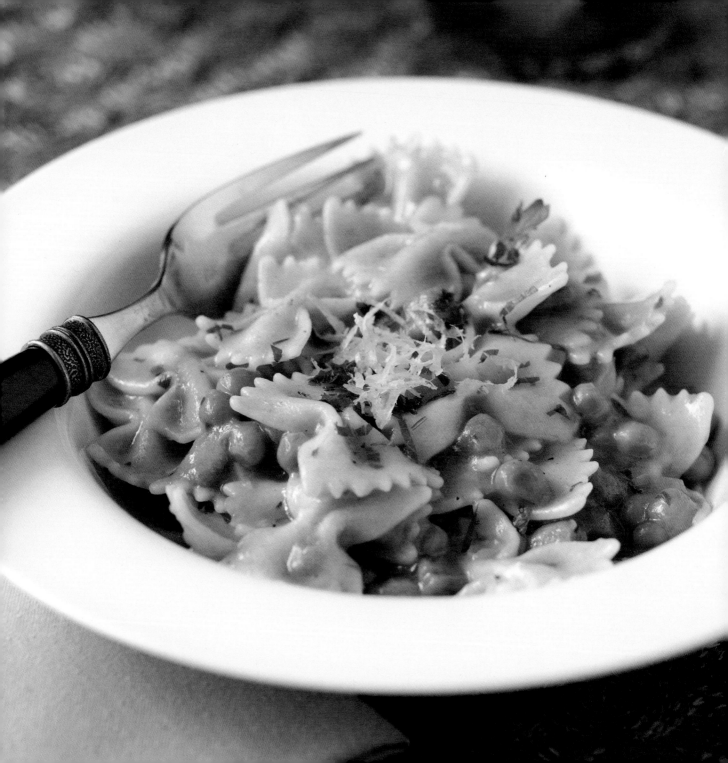

buttons and bows pasta

this light and lemon-y meal is a refreshing change to the same old pasta

2 C	dry whole-wheat bowtie pasta (farfalle) (8 oz)
1 Tbsp	olive oil
1 tsp	garlic, minced (about 1 clove)
1 bag	(16 oz) frozen peas and carrots
2 C	low-sodium chicken broth
2 Tbsp	cornstarch
1 Tbsp	fresh parsley, rinsed, dried, and chopped (or 1 tsp dried)
1	medium lemon, rinsed, for 1 tsp zest *(use a grater to take a thin layer of skin off the lemon)*
¼ tsp	ground black pepper

1. In a 4-quart saucepan, bring 3 quarts of water to a boil over high heat.
2. Add pasta, and cook according to package directions. Drain.
3. Meanwhile, heat olive oil and garlic over medium heat in a large sauté pan. Cook until soft, but not browned.
4. Add peas and carrots. Cook gently until the vegetables are heated through.
5. In a bowl, combine chicken broth and cornstarch. Mix well. Add to pan with vegetables, and bring to a boil. Simmer gently for 1 minute.
6. Add parsley, pasta, lemon zest, and pepper. Toss gently, and cook until the pasta is hot.
7. Serve 2 cups of pasta and vegetables per portion.

Note: Substitute cooking spray for olive oil and save calories and fat.

Children can help measure the dry pasta and mix ingredients together.

---

prep time:
5 minutes

cook time:
20 minutes

yield:
4 servings

serving size:
2 C pasta and vegetables

each serving provides:

calories	329	carbohydrates	59 g
total fat	6 g	potassium	331 mg
saturated fat	1 g	vitamin A	220%
cholesterol	0 mg	vitamin C	25%
sodium	127 mg	calcium	6%
total fiber	9 g	iron	10%
protein	13 g		

Percent Daily Values are based on a 2,000 calorie diet.

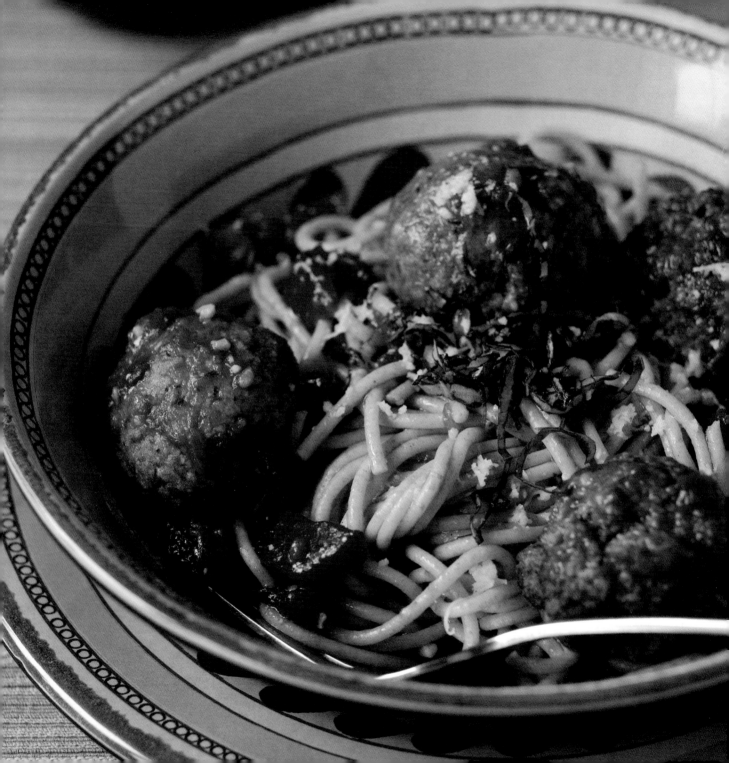

turkey and beef meatballs with whole-wheat spaghetti

HEALTHIER CLASSICS

easy and delicious—try serving with **Parmesan Green Beans** (on page 52)

8 oz	dry whole-wheat spaghetti
2 C	**Super Quick Chunky Tomato Sauce** *(see recipe on page 54)*
1 Tbsp	fresh basil, rinsed, dried, and chopped (or 1 tsp dried)
4 tsp	grated parmesan cheese

For turkey meatballs:

6 oz	99 percent lean ground turkey
¼ C	whole-wheat breadcrumbs
2 Tbsp	fat-free evaporated milk
1 Tbsp	grated parmesan cheese
½ Tbsp	fresh chives, rinsed, dried, and chopped (or 1 tsp dried)
½ Tbsp	fresh parsley, rinsed, dried, and chopped (or 1 tsp dried)

For beef meatballs:

6 oz	93 percent lean ground beef
¼ C	whole-wheat breadcrumbs
2 Tbsp	fat-free evaporated milk
1 Tbsp	grated parmesan cheese
½ Tbsp	fresh chives, rinsed, dried, and chopped (or 1 tsp dried)
½ Tbsp	fresh parsley, rinsed, dried, and chopped (or 1 tsp dried)

1. Preheat oven to 400 °F.
2. In a 4-quart saucepan, bring 3 quarts of water to a boil over high heat.
3. Add pasta, and cook according to package directions. Drain.
4. Meanwhile, combine ingredients for the turkey and beef meatballs in separate bowls, and mix well. Measure 1½ tablespoons of turkey mixture and roll in hand to form a ball; then place the meatball on a nonstick baking sheet. Repeat, and follow same instruction for beef mixture, until eight turkey and eight beef meatballs are made.
5. Bake meatballs on a nonstick baking sheet for 10 minutes (to a minimal internal temperature of 165 °F).
6. Warm sauce, if necessary.
7. Serve four meatballs, ¾ cup hot pasta, ½ cup sauce, 1 teaspoon cheese, and a pinch of basil per portion.

CHEFS IN TRAINING

Older children can help make the meatballs. Make sure everyone washes their hands and sanitizes all utensils and surfaces with disinfectant after handling raw meat.

prep time:
20 minutes
(25 minutes with homemade sauce)

cook time:
20 minutes
(35 minutes with homemade sauce)

yield:
4 servings

serving size:
4 meatballs, ¾ C pasta, ½ C sauce, 1 tsp cheese, pinch of basil

each serving provides:

calories	299	carbohydrates	37 g
total fat	5 g	potassium	194 mg
saturated fat	1 g	vitamin A	10%
cholesterol	41 mg	vitamin C	15%
sodium	277 mg	calcium	10%
total fiber	5 g	iron	25%
protein	28 g		

Percent Daily Values are based on a 2,000 calorie diet.

mediterranean pork penne

if this dish isn't simple enough for your children, see the tip below for serving "two ways"

2 C	dry whole-wheat penne pasta (8 oz)
1 Tbsp	olive oil
1 tsp	garlic, minced (about ½ clove)
8 oz	white button mushrooms, rinsed and cut into quarters
½ bag	(8 oz bag) sundried tomato halves, cut into thin strips
½ jar	(8 oz jar) artichoke hearts in water, drained, cut into quarters
2 C	low-sodium beef broth
2 Tbsp	cornstarch
12 oz	stir-fry pork strips, sliced into 12 strips (or, slice 3 4-oz boneless pork chops into thin strips)
¼ C	fat-free evaporated milk
2 Tbsp	fresh parsley, rinsed, dried, and chopped (or 2 tsp dried)

1. In a 4-quart saucepan, bring 3 quarts of water to a boil over high heat.
2. Add pasta, and cook according to package directions. Drain. (Set plain pasta aside for picky eaters—see Healthy Eating Two Ways suggestion below.)
3. Meanwhile, heat olive oil and garlic in a large sauté pan over medium heat. Cook until soft, but not browned (about 30 seconds).
4. Add mushrooms, and cook over medium heat until the mushrooms are soft and lightly browned.
5. Add sundried tomatoes and artichoke hearts. Toss gently to heat.
6. In a separate bowl, combine beef broth and cornstarch. Mix well.
7. Add broth mixture to the pan, and bring to a boil.
8. Add pork strips, evaporated milk, and parsley, and bring to a boil. Simmer gently for 3–5 minutes (to a minimum internal temperature of 160 °F).
9. Add pasta, and toss well to mix.
10. Serve 2 cups of pasta and sauce per portion.

For picky eaters, remove 3 ounces of pork from the pan and serve with ½ cup plain pasta and ½ cup steamed broccoli.

prep time: 10 minutes	**yield:** 4 servings	**each serving provides:**	
		calories	486
		total fat	11 g
cook time: 30 minutes	**serving size:** 2 C pasta and sauce	saturated fat	3 g
		cholesterol	50 mg
		sodium	250 mg
		total fiber	8 g
		protein	33 g

each serving provides:

calories	486	carbohydrates	56 g
total fat	11 g	potassium	790 mg
saturated fat	3 g	vitamin A	15%
cholesterol	50 mg	vitamin C	15%
sodium	250 mg	calcium	10%
total fiber	8 g	iron	25%
protein	33 g		

Percent Daily Values are based on a 2,000 calorie diet.

bowtie pasta with chicken, broccoli, and feta

this yummy dish provides a tasty way to get your children to eat broccoli

2 C	dry whole-wheat bowtie pasta (farfalle) (8 oz)
1 Tbsp	olive oil
1 tsp	garlic, minced (about ½ clove)
8 oz	white button mushrooms, rinsed and cut into quarters
4 C	cooked broccoli florets (or 1 1-lb bag frozen broccoli, thawed)
1 C	grilled boneless, skinless chicken breast, diced (about 2 small breasts) *(Leftover Friendly)*
2 C	low-sodium chicken broth
1	medium lemon, rinsed, for 1 tsp zest and 1 Tbsp juice *(use a grater to take a thin layer of skin off the lemon; squeeze juice and set aside)*
2 oz	reduced-fat feta cheese, diced *(Healthy Eating Two Ways)*

1. In a 4-quart saucepan, bring 3 quarts of water to a boil over high heat.
2. Add pasta, and cook according to package directions. Drain.
3. Heat olive oil and garlic in a large sauté pan over medium heat. Cook until soft, but not browned (about 30 seconds).
4. Add mushrooms and heat until lightly browned and soft.
5. Add broccoli, diced chicken, and chicken broth. Bring to a boil and simmer for about 3 minutes, until the broccoli and chicken are heated through.
6. Add pasta, and toss gently. Continue to simmer until pasta is hot, about 3–4 minutes.
7. Add lemon zest and juice, and toss gently.
8. Serve 2 cups of pasta and sauce per portion. Top each portion with 1½ tablespoons feta cheese.

If you don't have leftover cooked chicken, see basic cooking instructions in appendix D (page 103).

If your children do not like feta cheese, try serving with parmesan or mozzarella cheese on top.

prep time:
15 minutes

cook time:
15 minutes

yield:
4 servings

serving size:
1 C pasta, 1 C sauce, 1½ Tbsp feta

each serving provides:

calories	421	carbohydrates	49 g
total fat	10 g	potassium	697 mg
saturated fat	2 g	vitamin A	30%
cholesterol	65 mg	vitamin C	140%
sodium	285 mg	calcium	10%
total fiber	8 g	iron	10%
protein	36 g		

Percent Daily Values are based on a 2,000 calorie diet.

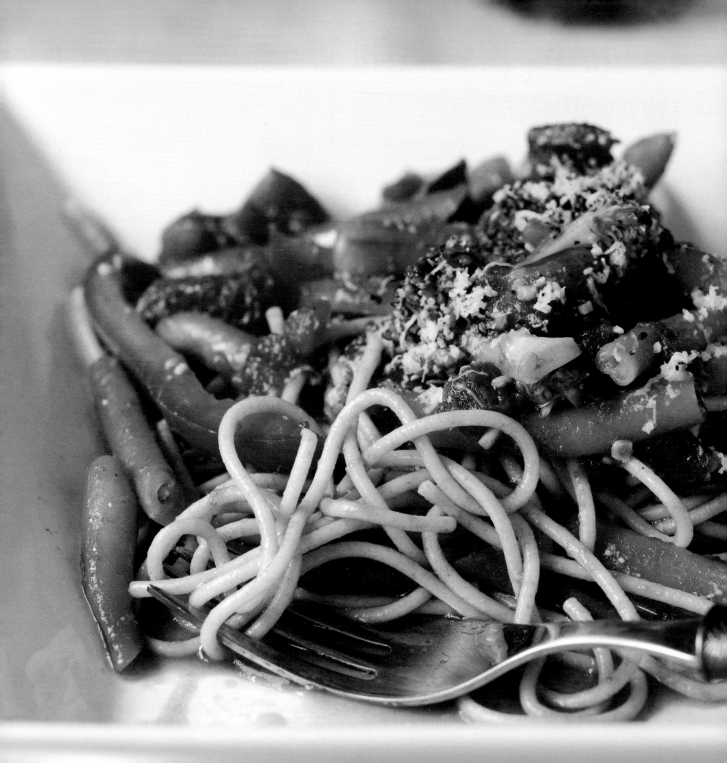

pasta primavera

pasta, vegetables, and a sprinkle of cheese make this a child-friendly classic that adults will love too

8 oz	dry whole-wheat spaghetti
1 Tbsp	olive oil
1 tsp	garlic, minced (about ½ clove)
4 C	assorted cooked vegetables— such as red pepper strips, broccoli florets, carrot sticks, or green beans (*Leftover Friendly*)
1 can	(15½ oz) no-salt-added diced tomatoes
1 can	(5½ oz) low-sodium tomato juice
¼ tsp	ground black pepper
¼ C	grated parmesan cheese

1. In a 4-quart saucepan, bring 3 quarts of water to a boil over high heat.

2. Add spaghetti, and cook according to package directions. Drain.

3. Meanwhile, combine olive oil and garlic in a large sauté pan. Cook until garlic is soft, but not browned (about 30 seconds).

4. Add mixed vegetables, and cook until vegetables are soft, but not browned (about 3–5 minutes).

5. Add diced tomatoes, tomato juice, and pepper. Bring to a boil. Reduce heat, and simmer for 5 minutes.

6. Add spaghetti and parmesan cheese. Toss until the pasta is hot and well mixed, and serve.

pasta dishes

Note: Substitute cooking spray for olive oil and save calories and fat.

If you don't have leftover cooked vegetables, see basic cooking instructions in appendix D (page 103).

prep time:	yield:	each serving provides:			
5 minutes	4 servings	calories	319	carbohydrates	59 g
		total fat	6 g	potassium	596 mg
cook time:	serving size:	saturated fat	2 g	vitamin A	140%
20 minutes	2 C pasta and vegetables	cholesterol	4 mg	vitamin C	160%
		sodium	167 mg	calcium	15%
		total fiber	12 g	iron	20%
		protein	13 g		

Percent Daily Values are based on a 2,000 calorie diet.

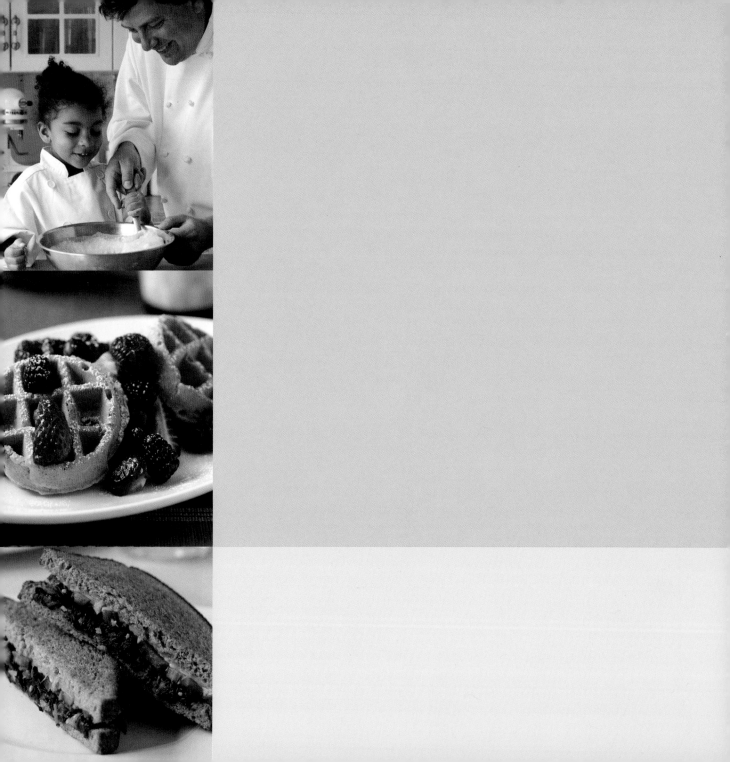

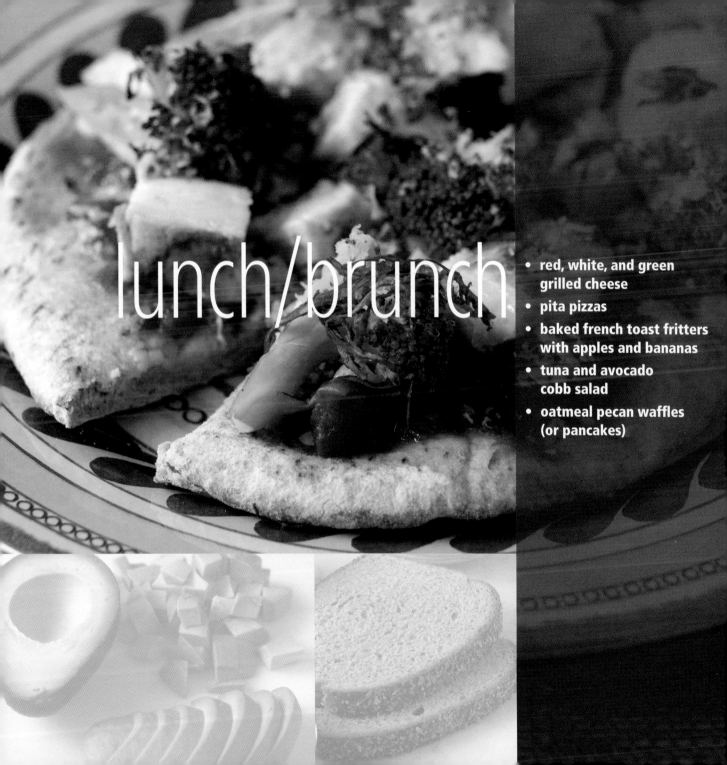

lunch/brunch

- red, white, and green grilled cheese
- pita pizzas
- baked french toast fritters with apples and bananas
- tuna and avocado cobb salad
- oatmeal pecan waffles (or pancakes)

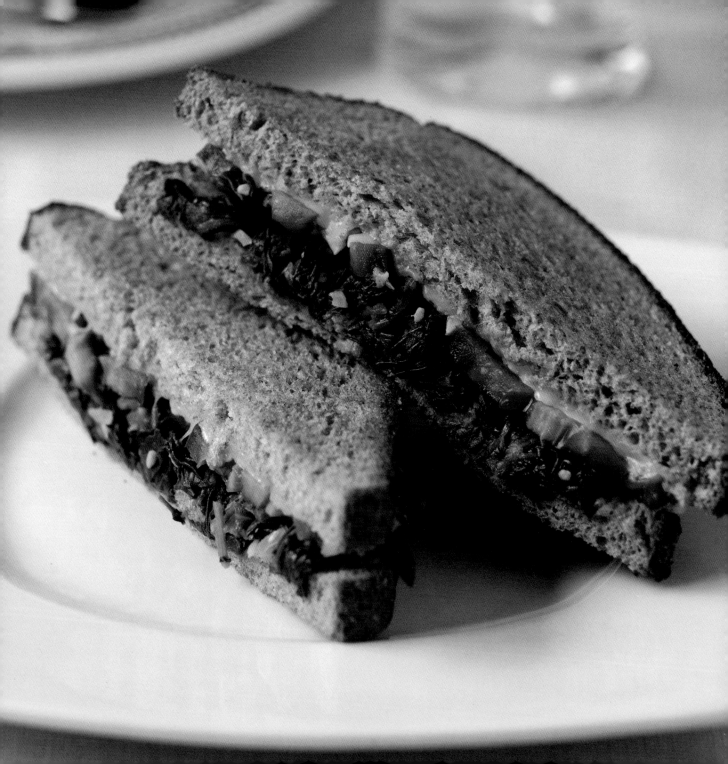

red, white, and green grilled cheese

so good, your children might not even notice the "green stuff"

1 tsp	garlic, minced (about ½ clove)
1	small onion, minced (about ½ cup)
2 C	frozen cut spinach, thawed and drained *(or substitute 2 bags (10 oz each) fresh leaf spinach, rinsed)*
¼ tsp	ground black pepper
8 slices	whole-wheat bread
1	medium tomato, rinsed, cut into 4 slices
1 C	shredded part-skim mozzarella cheese
Nonstick cooking spray	

1. Preheat oven to 400 °F. Place a large baking sheet in the oven to preheat for about 10 minutes.

2. Heat garlic with cooking spray in a medium sauté pan over medium heat. Cook until soft, but not browned. Add onions, and continue to cook until the onions are soft, but not browned.

3. Add spinach, and toss gently. Cook until the spinach is heated throughout. Season with pepper, and set aside to cool.

4. When the spinach and onions are cool, assemble each sandwich with one slice of bread on the bottom, one tomato slice, ½ cup of spinach mixture, ¼ cup of cheese, and a second slice of bread on the top. (For picky eaters, see Healthy Eating Two Ways suggestion below.)

5. Spray the preheated nonstick baking sheet with cooking spray. Place the sandwiches on the baking sheet. Bake for 10 minutes, or until the bottom of each sandwich is browned.

6. Carefully flip sandwiches, and bake for an additional 5 minutes, or until both sides are browned. Serve immediately.

 For picky eaters, start with less spinach in the sandwich, and possibly serve the remaining amount on the side.

prep time: 15 minutes	**yield:** 4 servings	
cook time: 15 minutes	**serving size:** 1 sandwich	

each serving provides:

calories	254	carbohydrates	29 g
total fat	8 g	potassium	364 mg
saturated fat	4 g	vitamin A	130%
cholesterol	18 mg	vitamin C	6%
sodium	468 mg	calcium	35%
total fiber	6 g	iron	15%
protein	17 g		

Percent Daily Values are based on a 2,000 calorie diet.

lunch/brunch

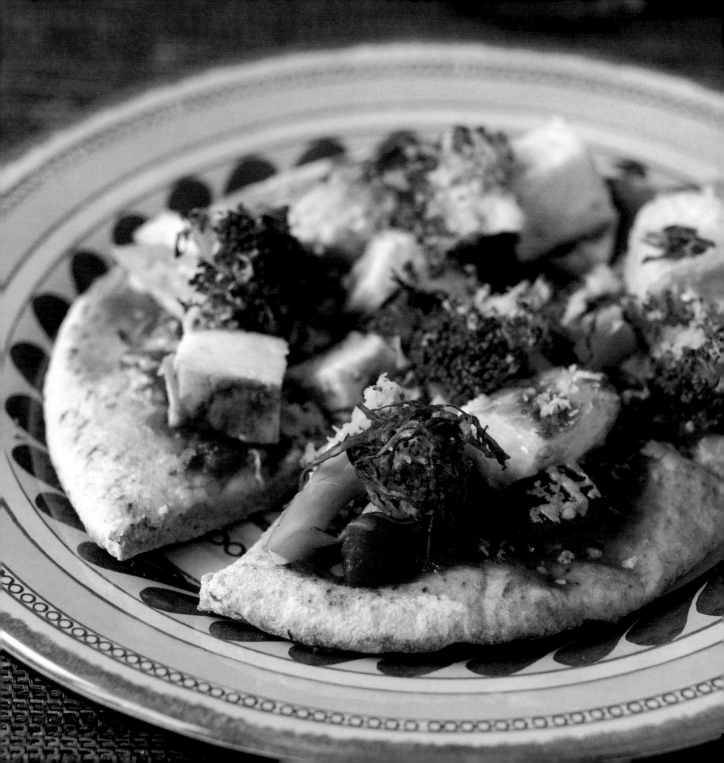

pita pizzas

personal pita pizzas are fun to make, and even more fun to eat!

1 C	**Super Quick Chunky Tomato Sauce** *(see recipe on page 54)*
1 C	**grilled boneless, skinless chicken breast, diced (about 2 small breasts)**
1 C	**broccoli, rinsed, chopped, and cooked**
2 Tbsp	**grated parmesan cheese**
1 Tbsp	**fresh basil, rinsed, dried, and chopped (or 1 tsp dried)**
4	**(6½-inch) whole-wheat pitas**

1. Preheat oven or toaster oven to 450 °F.
2. For each pizza, spread ¼ cup tomato sauce on a pita and top with ¼ cup chicken, ¼ cup broccoli, ½ tablespoon parmesan cheese, and ¼ tablespoon chopped basil.
3. Place pitas on a nonstick baking sheet and bake for about 5–8 minutes until golden brown and chicken is heated through. Serve immediately.

Keep ingredients on hand for older children to make pita pizzas for themselves. Younger children can help top their own personal pizzas.

prep time:
10 minutes
(15 minutes with homemade sauce)

cook time:
8 minutes
(23 minutes with homemade sauce)

yield:
4 servings

serving size:
1 pita pizza

each serving provides:

calories	275	carbohydrates	41 g
total fat	5 g	potassium	362 mg
saturated fat	1 g	vitamin A	15%
cholesterol	32 mg	vitamin C	50%
sodium	486 mg	calcium	10%
total fiber	7 g	iron	15%
protein	20 g		

Percent Daily Values are based on a 2,000 calorie diet.

baked french toast fritters with apples and bananas

add fruit to your meal with this heavenly, melt-in-your-mouth dish

For sandwiches:

8 slices	whole-wheat bread
¼ C	creamy peanut butter (or other nut butter)
1	apple, rinsed, peeled, cored, and sliced into 8 rings
2	bananas, peeled and cut into about 12 thin slices each

For batter:

3 Tbsp	egg substitute (or substitute 1 egg white)
¼ tsp	ground cinnamon
1 Tbsp	brown sugar
¼ C	fat-free evaporated milk

Nonstick cooking spray

1. Preheat oven to 400 °F. Place a large baking sheet in the oven to preheat for about 10 minutes.
2. Assemble fritter as a sandwich, with ½ tablespoon of peanut butter on each slice of bread, and two apple slices and six banana slices in the middle of each sandwich.
3. Combine ingredients for the batter, and mix well.
4. Spray a nonstick baking sheet with cooking spray.
5. Dip both sides of each fritter in the batter, and place fritters on preheated baking sheet. Bake for 10 minutes on each side, or until both sides are browned. Serve immediately.

Children can help slice the apples and bananas and spread the peanut butter.

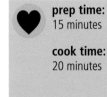

prep time: 15 minutes	**yield:** 4 servings		
cook time: 20 minutes	**serving size:** 1 fritter		

each serving provides:

calories	332	carbohydrates	50 g
total fat	10 g	potassium	543 mg
saturated fat	2 g	vitamin A	4%
cholesterol	0 mg	vitamin C	2%
sodium	374 mg	calcium	10%
total fiber	7 g	iron	15%
protein	14 g		

Percent Daily Values are based on a 2,000 calorie diet.

tuna and avocado cobb salad

not just a salad, but a delicious meal—try serving with crusty whole-grain bread

For salad:

4 C	red leaf lettuce, rinsed and chopped (about 8 leaves)
1 C	frozen whole kernel corn, roasted *(on a pan in the oven or toaster oven at 400 °F for 7–10 minutes)*
1 C	carrots, shredded
1	tomato, rinsed, halved and sliced
½	ripe avocado, peeled and sliced*
1 C	frozen green peas, thawed
1 can	(6 oz) canned white albacore tuna in water

For dressing:

2 Tbsp	lemon juice (or about 1 fresh lemon)
1 Tbsp	lime juice (or about 1 fresh lime)
1 Tbsp	honey
1 Tbsp	fresh parsley, rinsed, dried, and minced (or 1 tsp dried)
1 Tbsp	water
1 Tbsp	olive oil

1. Divide and arrange 2 cups of salad ingredients in each of 4 serving bowls.
2. For dressing, combine all ingredients and mix well. Spoon 2 tablespoons over each salad, and serve.

Tip: Look for an avocado that is slightly firm, but soft enough to be gently squeezed. For a description of how to peel and cut an avocado, see the FAQs in appendix D (on page 106).

Note: Four ounces of fresh grilled tuna steaks, salmon, or shrimp can be substituted for the albacore tuna. For cooking instructions for fresh fish and shellfish, see basic cooking instructions in appendix D (on page 103).

* Use the other half of the avocado for the **Quinoa-Stuffed Tomatoes** (on page 58).

lunch/brunch

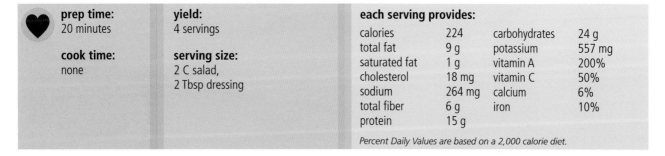

prep time: 20 minutes	**yield:** 4 servings	**each serving provides:**	
		calories	224	carbohydrates	24 g

each serving provides:			
calories	224	carbohydrates	24 g
total fat	9 g	potassium	557 mg
saturated fat	1 g	vitamin A	200%
cholesterol	18 mg	vitamin C	50%
sodium	264 mg	calcium	6%
total fiber	6 g	iron	10%
protein	15 g		

prep time: 20 minutes

cook time: none

yield: 4 servings

serving size: 2 C salad, 2 Tbsp dressing

Percent Daily Values are based on a 2,000 calorie diet.

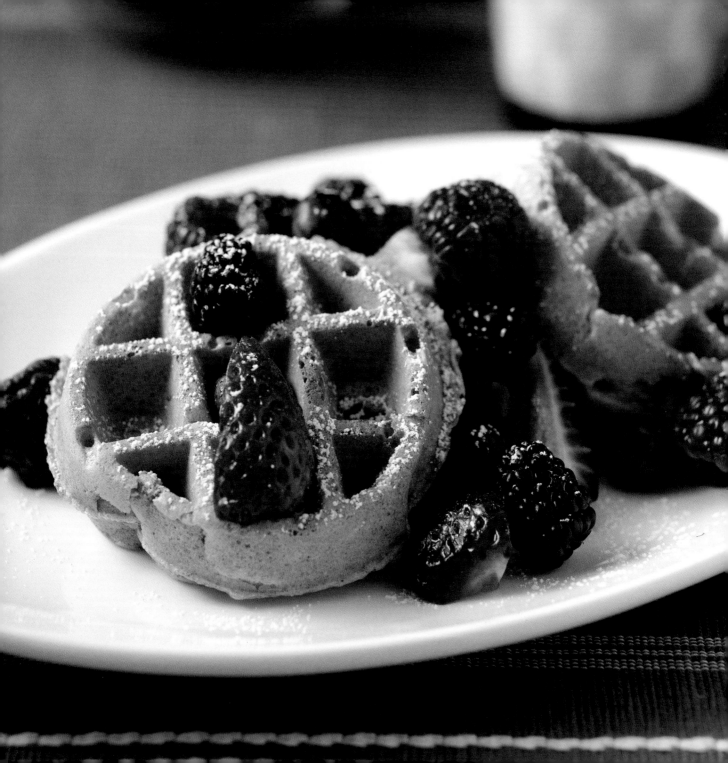

oatmeal pecan waffles (or pancakes)

your children will jump right out of bed for this delicious meal

For waffles:

1 C	whole-wheat flour
½ C	quick-cooking oats
2 tsp	baking powder
1 tsp	sugar
¼ C	unsalted pecans, chopped
2	large eggs, separated *(for pancakes, see note)*
1½ C	fat-free (skim) milk
1 Tbsp	vegetable oil

For fruit topping:

2 C	fresh strawberries, rinsed, stems removed, and cut in half *(or substitute frozen strawberries, thawed)*
1 C	fresh blackberries, rinsed *(or substitute frozen blackberries, thawed)*
1 C	fresh blueberries, rinsed *(or substitute frozen blueberries, thawed)*
1 tsp	powdered sugar

1. Preheat waffle iron.
2. Combine flour, oats, baking powder, sugar, and pecans in a large bowl.
3. Combine egg yolks, milk, and vegetable oil in a separate bowl, and mix well.
4. Add liquid mixture to the dry ingredients, and stir together. Do not overmix; mixture should be a bit lumpy.
5. Whip egg whites to medium peaks. Gently fold egg whites into batter (for pancakes, see note below).
6. Pour batter into preheated waffle iron, and cook until the waffle iron light signals it's done or steam stops coming out of the iron. (A waffle is perfect when it is crisp and well-browned on the outside with a moist, light, airy and fluffy inside.) *(Batter also can be used to make pancakes; see note below.)*
7. Add fresh fruit and a light dusting of powdered sugar to each waffle, and serve.

Note: For pancakes, do not separate eggs. Mix whole eggs with milk and oil, and eliminate steps 4 and 5.

Children can mix the batter and top each waffle/pancake with fruit.

lunch/brunch

prep time: 10 minutes	**yield:** 4 servings	**each serving provides:**	
		calories	340	carbohydrates	50 g
		total fat	11 g	potassium	369 mg
cook time: 30 minutes	**serving size:** 3 small (2-inch) or 1 large (6-inch) waffle (depending on waffle iron size) or pancakes	saturated fat	2 g	vitamin A	8%
		cholesterol	107 mg	vitamin C	60%
		sodium	331 mg	calcium	30%
		total fiber	9 g	iron	6%
		protein	14 g		

Percent Daily Values are based on a 2,000 calorie diet.

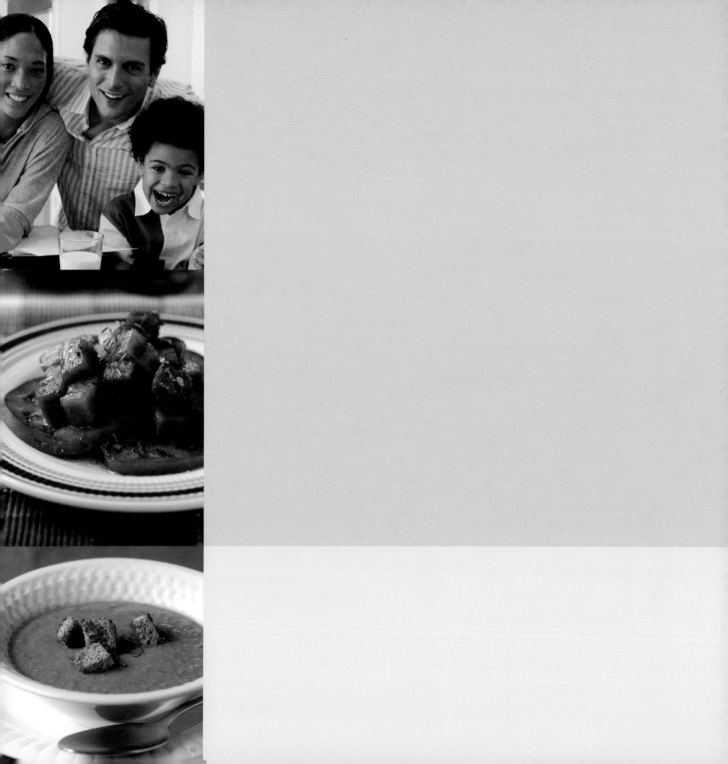

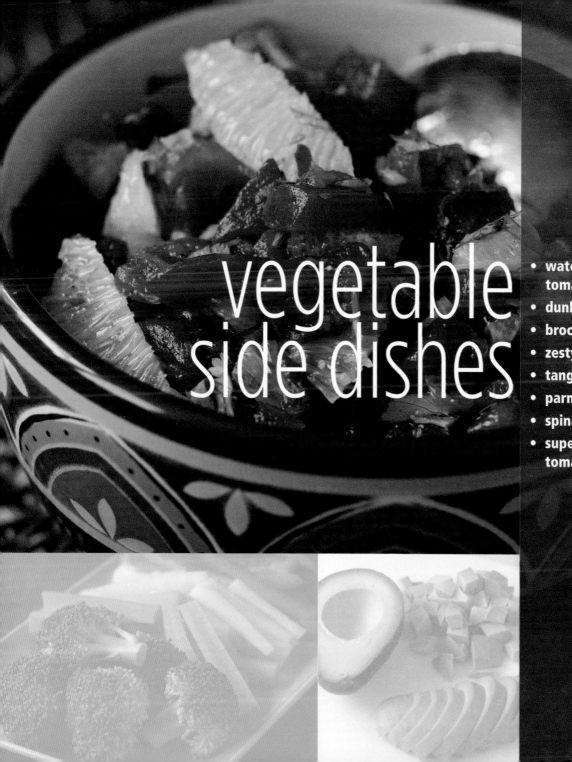

vegetable
side dishes

- **watermelon and tomato salad**
- **dunkin' veggies and dips**
- **broccoli and cheese**
- **zesty tomato soup**
- **tangy salsa**
- **parmesan green beans**
- **spinach and corn pancakes**
- **super quick chunky tomato sauce**

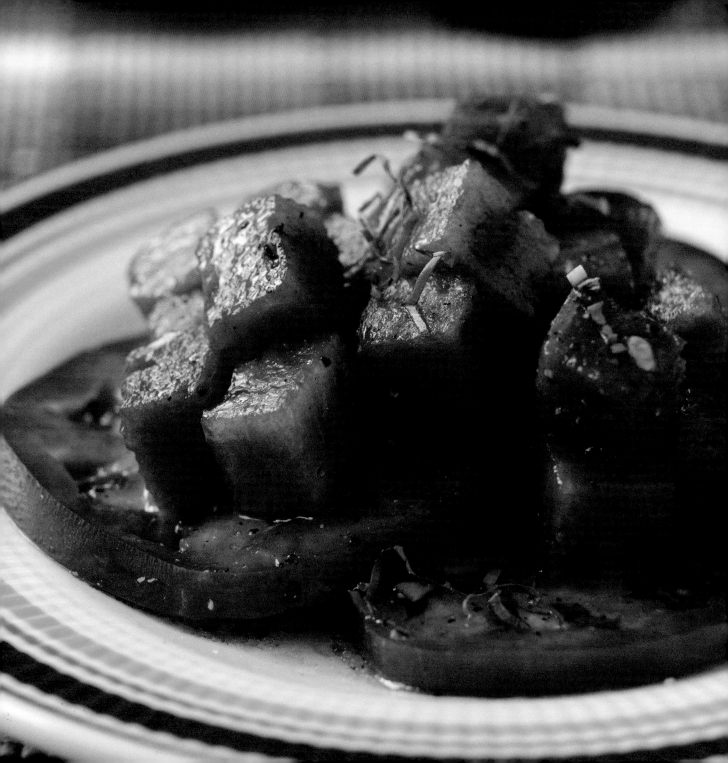

watermelon and tomato salad

a perfect mixture of tangy and sweet

2	large tomatoes, rinsed and cut into 6 slices each
2 Tbsp	white balsamic vinegar *(or substitute apple cider vinegar)*
1 Tbsp	olive oil
1 Tbsp	fresh basil, rinsed, dried, and chopped (or 1 tsp dried)
4 C	diced watermelon, with seeds removed (about half a small melon, rinsed)
¼ tsp	salt
¼ tsp	ground black pepper

1. Arrange three tomato slices on each of four salad plates.
2. Combine vinegar, oil, and basil in a bowl, and mix well.
3. Add watermelon, and gently toss to coat evenly.
4. Spoon watermelon over the tomatoes.
5. Top with salt and pepper, and serve.

 Substitute three cherry or grape tomatoes and three chunks of watermelon threaded onto a wooden skewer (eight skewers needed). Serving: two skewers.

 Children can help mix the salad or thread the skewers.

prep time:	yield:	each serving provides:			
20 minutes	4 servings	calories	96	carbohydrates	16 g
		total fat	4 g	potassium	390 mg
cook time:	serving size:	saturated fat	1 g	vitamin A	35%
none	3 tomato slices, 1 C watermelon (or 2 skewers)	cholesterol	0 mg	vitamin C	40%
		sodium	127 mg	calcium	2%
		total fiber	2 g	iron	10%
		protein	2 g		

Percent Daily Values are based on a 2,000 calorie diet.

vegetable side dishes

dunkin' veggies and dips

dipping makes veggies fun—try these tasty dips for dinner, a snack, or a party!

Low-fat blue cheese dip:

¼ C	reduced-fat blue cheese crumbles
¼ C	fat-free sour cream
2 Tbsp	light mayonnaise

Honey mustard dip:

¼ C	honey
2 Tbsp	brown mustard
2 Tbsp	fat-free evaporated milk
1 Tbsp	fresh parsley, rinsed, dried, and chopped (or 1 tsp dried)
1 Tbsp	fresh chives, rinsed, dried, and chopped (or 1 tsp dried)

Tuscan white bean dip:

1 Tbsp	olive oil
1 Tbsp	garlic, chopped (about 3 cloves)
2 Tbsp	onions, chopped
1 C	low-sodium cannellini beans, rinsed
¼ C	low-sodium chicken broth
1 Tbsp	fresh parsley, rinsed, dried, and chopped (or 1 tsp dried)
1 tsp	fresh oregano, rinsed, dried, and chopped (or ¼ tsp dried)

Vegetables:

5 C	assorted raw vegetables, rinsed and cut into bite-sized pieces as needed—such as baby carrots, celery sticks, broccoli florets, cauliflower florets, or cherry tomatoes

1. Combine ingredients for any (or all) of these three dips separately, and set aside (see note below).
2. Arrange vegetables on a platter, and serve with choice of dip.

continued on page 45

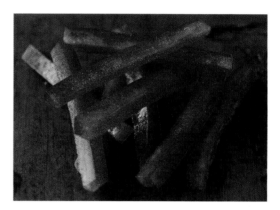

Note: Tuscan white bean dip requires a mixer, masher, or big spoon to make the dip smooth. If you can't find beans that are labeled "low sodium," compare the Nutrition Facts panels to find the beans with the lowest amount of sodium. Rinsing can help reduce sodium levels further.

CHEFS IN TRAINING

Children can help make the dips and rinse the vegetables.

prep time: 5–10 minutes for each dip	**yield:** 4 servings
cook time: none	**serving size:** 1 Tbsp dip (nutrients listed separately for each dip and for 1½ C vegetables)

dunkin' veggies and dips (continued)

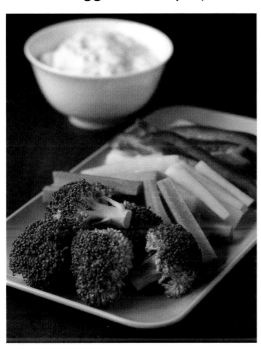

each serving provides:

low-fat blue cheese dip (1 Tbsp):

calories	56	carbohydrates	3 g
total fat	4 g	potassium	22 mg
saturated fat	1 g	vitamin A	2%
cholesterol	4 mg	vitamin C	0%
sodium	145 mg	calcium	2%
total fiber	0 g	iron	0%
protein	3 g		

honey mustard dip (1 Tbsp):

calories	71	carbohydrates	19 g
total fat	0 g	potassium	86 mg
saturated fat	0 g	vitamin A	4%
cholesterol	0 mg	vitamin C	4%
sodium	46 mg	calcium	2%
total fiber	0 g	iron	0%
protein	1 g		

tuscan white bean dip (1 Tbsp):

calories	87	carbohydrates	10 g
total fat	4 g	potassium	158 mg
saturated fat	1 g	vitamin A	2%
cholesterol	0 mg	vitamin C	4%
sodium	25 mg	calcium	0%
total fiber	3 g	iron	6%
protein	3 g		

vegetables (1½ C mixed baby carrots, celery sticks, broccoli florets, cauliflower florets, or cherry tomatoes):

calories	42	carbohydrates	9 g
total fat	0 g	potassium	456 mg
saturated fat	0 g	vitamin A	140%
cholesterol	0 mg	vitamin C	80%
sodium	77 mg	calcium	6%
total fiber	2 g	iron	10%
protein	2 g		

Percent Daily Values are based on a 2,000 calorie diet.

vegetable side dishes

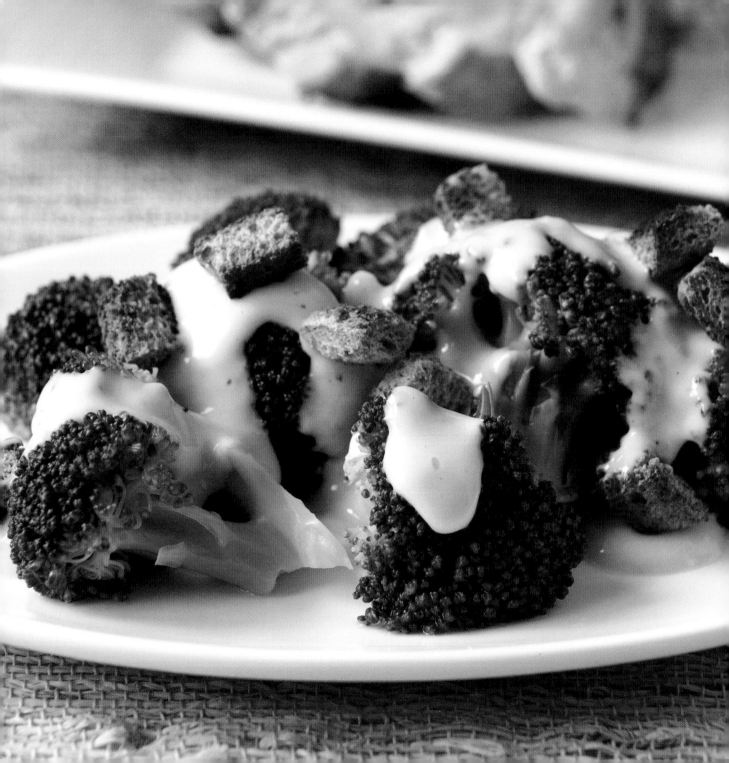

broccoli and cheese

so good, your children will ask for seconds—and a perfect side for most chicken and beef dishes

6 C	fresh broccoli, rinsed and cut into bite-sized florets *(or substitute 6 C frozen broccoli, thawed and warmed, and skip step 1)*

For sauce:

1 C	fat-free evaporated milk
1 Tbsp	cornstarch
½ C	shredded cheddar cheese
¼ tsp	Worcestershire sauce
¼ tsp	hot sauce
1 slice	whole-wheat bread, diced and toasted (for croutons)*

1. Bring a large pot of water to boil over high heat. Add fresh broccoli, and cook until easily pierced by a fork, about 7–10 minutes. Drain and set aside.
2. In a separate saucepan, combine evaporated milk and cornstarch. Slowly bring to a boil while stirring often.
3. When the milk comes to a boil, remove it from the heat and add the cheese. Continue to stir until the cheese is melted and evenly mixed.
4. Add the Worcestershire and hot sauces, and stir.
5. Pour cheese over hot broccoli.
6. Sprinkle whole-wheat croutons over broccoli and cheese mixture, and serve.

* Make extra croutons for the **Zesty Tomato Soup** (on page 49).

Children can help measure ingredients and mix the sauce.

vegetable side dishes

prep time:
15 minutes

cook time:
15 minutes

yield:
4 servings

serving size:
1½ C broccoli,
¼ C sauce,
1 Tbsp croutons

each serving provides:

calories	162	carbohydrates	19 g
total fat	5 g	potassium	601 mg
saturated fat	3 g	vitamin A	70%
cholesterol	15 mg	vitamin C	170%
sodium	239 mg	calcium	30%
total fiber	4 g	iron	8%
protein	11 g		

Percent Daily Values are based on a 2,000 calorie diet.

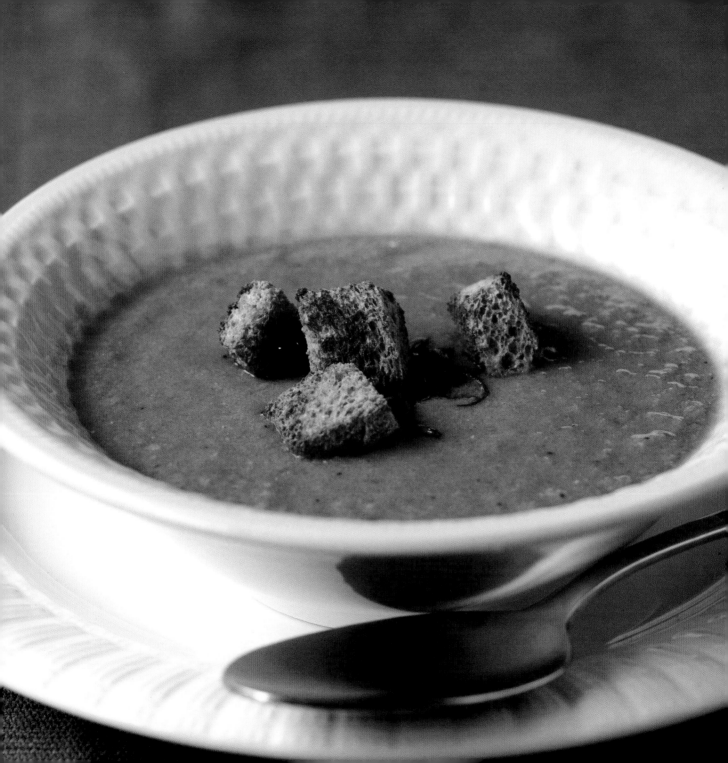

zesty tomato soup

not your traditional tomato soup, this quick-cooking dish can be a side or light main meal

1 can	**(14½ oz) no-salt-added diced tomatoes**
1 C	**jarred roasted red peppers, drained** *(or substitute fresh roasted red peppers; see tip)*
1 C	**fat-free evaporated milk**
1 tsp	**garlic powder**
¼ tsp	**ground black pepper**
2 Tbsp	**fresh basil, rinsed and chopped (or 2 tsp dried)**

1. Combine tomatoes and red peppers in a blender or food processor. Puree until smooth.
2. Put tomato mixture in a medium saucepan, and bring to a boil over medium heat.
3. Add evaporated milk, garlic powder, and pepper. Return to a boil, and gently simmer for 5 minutes.
4. Add basil, and serve.
5. Optional step: Serve with whole-wheat croutons sprinkled on top (from **Broccoli and Cheese,** page 47).

Tip: To make roasted red peppers, see instructions in the FAQs in appendix D (on page 108). Make extra to use in other Keep the Beat™ recipes.

Older children can make the recipe themselves.

vegetable side dishes

prep time:
10 minutes

cook time:
15 minutes

yield:
4 servings

serving size:
1 C soup

each serving provides:

calories	94	carbohydrates	16 g
total fat	0 g	potassium	234 mg
saturated fat	0 g	vitamin A	15%
cholesterol	0 mg	vitamin C	15%
sodium	231 mg	calcium	0%
total fiber	2 g	iron	2%
protein	5 g		

Percent Daily Values are based on a 2,000 calorie diet.

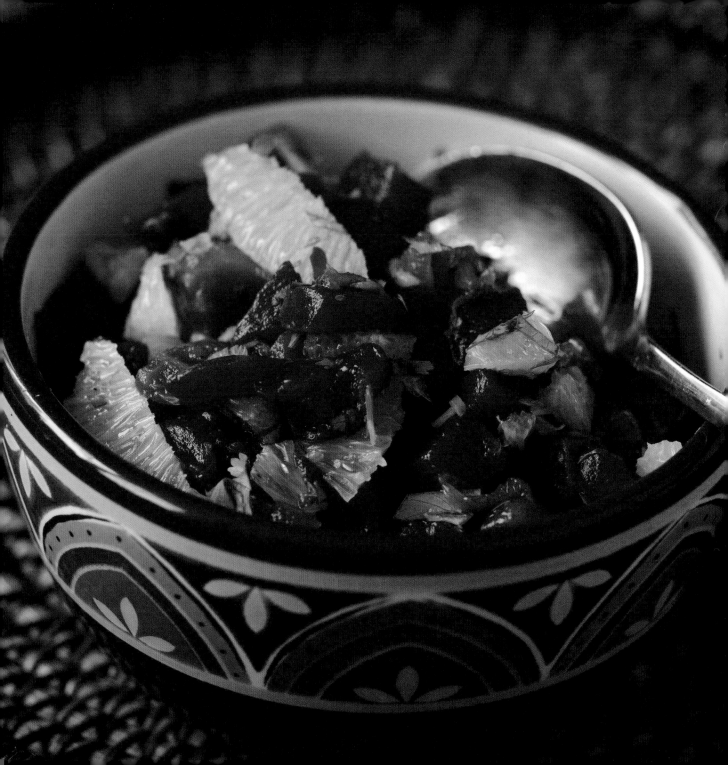

tangy salsa

tangy, not spicy, this salsa will appeal to most—try it with the **Empañapita** (on page 7) or as a dip with veggies or baked chips

½ C	jarred roasted red peppers, drained and diced *(or substitute fresh roasted red peppers; see tip) (Leftover Friendly)*
½ C	no-salt-added diced tomatoes *(or substitute 1 medium tomato, chopped)*
1	small lime, peeled and cut into small chunks
¼ tsp	ground black pepper
¼ tsp	ground cumin
1 Tbsp	fresh cilantro, rinsed and chopped *(or substitute 1 tsp dried coriander)*

1. Combine all ingredients, and toss well.
2. Best to allow 1–2 hours for flavors to settle before serving.

Tip: To make roasted red peppers, see instructions in the FAQs in appendix D (on page 108). Make extra to use in other Keep the Beat™ recipes.

 Substitute fresh roasted red peppers by making extra when you make the **Super Quick Chunky Tomato Sauce** (on page 54). If you don't have leftover cooked vegetables, see basic cooking instructions in appendix D (page 103).

vegetable side dishes

prep time: 10 minutes	**yield:** 4 servings	**each serving provides:**			
		calories	23	carbohydrates	4 g
cook time: none	**serving size:** ¼ C salsa	total fat	0 g	potassium	18 mg
		saturated fat	0 g	vitamin A	4%
		cholesterol	0 mg	vitamin C	10%
		sodium	68 mg	calcium	2%
		total fiber	1 g	iron	2%
		protein	0 g		

Percent Daily Values are based on a 2,000 calorie diet.

parmesan green beans

a side dish so tasty, children won't even know it's good for them

1 Tbsp	olive oil
1 tsp	garlic, minced (about 1 clove) (or ¼ tsp garlic powder)
1	small onion, thinly sliced (about ½ C)
1 bag	(16 oz) frozen green beans
1 C	low-sodium chicken broth
¼ C	grated parmesan cheese
¼ tsp	ground black pepper

1. Combine olive oil and garlic in a large saucepan. Cook until garlic is soft, but not browned (about 30 seconds).
2. Add onion, and continue to cook for about 5 minutes over medium heat until soft.
3. Add green beans and chicken broth. Bring to a boil and simmer for 2 minutes, until the beans are heated through.
4. Sprinkle with parmesan cheese and pepper, and serve.

Tip: Try it on the side of the **Turkey and Beef Meatballs With Whole-Wheat Spaghetti** (on page 25).

 Children can help sprinkle with cheese and pepper.

prep time:	yield:	each serving provides:			
5 minutes	4 servings	calories	95	carbohydrates	9 g
		total fat	5 g	potassium	293 mg
cook time:	serving size:	saturated fat	1 g	vitamin A	15%
8 minutes	1 C green bean mix	cholesterol	4 mg	vitamin C	25%
		sodium	117 mg	calcium	10%
		total fiber	3 g	iron	4%
		protein	5 g		

Percent Daily Values are based on a 2,000 calorie diet.

spinach and corn pancakes

vegetables in a pancake? serve this fun side dish with most chicken, meat, or fish dishes

½ C	whole-wheat flour
1 C	fat-free (skim) milk
2 Tbsp	vegetable oil
2	large eggs
1 C	frozen chopped spinach, thawed and drained
1 C	frozen whole corn kernels, thawed
¼ tsp	ground black pepper
Nonstick cooking spray	

1. Measure flour into a large mixing bowl.
2. In a smaller bowl, combine milk, oil, and eggs, and mix well. Add milk mixture to flour, and mix until smooth.
3. Add spinach, corn, and pepper to mixture, and stir well.
4. Heat a large nonstick sauté pan or griddle. Spray lightly with cooking spray.
5. Spoon batter ¼ cup at a time onto the pan. Cook each pancake for 2–3 minutes, or until the bottom holds together and is golden brown. Carefully flip and cook the second side for an additional 1–2 minutes. (Recipe makes about 16–18 pancakes.)
6. Serve immediately.

Older children can help mix the ingredients and flip the pancakes.

prep time: 10 minutes	**yield:** 4 servings	**each serving provides:**			
		calories	227	carbohydrates	27 g
cook time: 25 minutes	**serving size:** about 4 pancakes	total fat	10 g	potassium	391 mg
		saturated fat	2 g	vitamin A	110%
		cholesterol	107 mg	vitamin C	30%
		sodium	128 mg	calcium	15%
		total fiber	4 g	iron	15%
		protein	11 g		

Percent Daily Values are based on a 2,000 calorie diet.

vegetable side dishes

super quick chunky tomato sauce
make batches of this tasty sauce to go with a number of recipes in this cookbook

2 tsp	olive oil
1 tsp	garlic, chopped (about 1 clove)
1 jar	(12 oz) roasted red peppers, drained and diced (or substitute fresh roasted red peppers; see tip)
2 cans	(14½ oz each) no-salt-added diced tomatoes
1 can	(5½ oz) low-sodium tomato juice
1 Tbsp	fresh basil, rinsed, dried, and chopped (or 1 tsp dried)
¼ tsp	ground black pepper

1. In a medium saucepan, heat olive oil and garlic over medium heat. Cook until soft, but not browned (for about 30 seconds).

2. Add diced red peppers, and continue to cook for 2–3 minutes, until the peppers begin to sizzle.

3. Add tomatoes, tomato juice, basil, and pepper. Bring to a boil. Simmer for 10 minutes, or until the sauce thickens slightly. (Sauce can be pureed for picky eaters.)

4. Use immediately. Or, refrigerate in a tightly sealed container for 3–5 days or freeze for 1–2 months.

Tip: To make roasted red peppers, see instructions in the FAQs in appendix D (on page 108). Make extra to use in other Keep the Beat™ recipes.

Older children can chop the roasted red peppers and help cook the sauce. For a delicious change, try making fresh roasted red peppers.

prep time: 5 minutes	**yield:** 12 servings	
cook time: 15 minutes (add 15 minutes if making homemade roasted red peppers)	**serving size:** ½ C sauce	

each serving provides:

calories	31	carbohydrates	4 g
total fat	1 g	potassium	66 mg
saturated fat	0 g	vitamin A	6%
cholesterol	0 mg	vitamin C	15%
sodium	76 mg	calcium	2%
total fiber	1 g	iron	2%
protein	1 g		

Percent Daily Values are based on a 2,000 calorie diet.

grain side dishes

- roasted red pepper and toasted orzo
- wow-y maui pasta salad
- quinoa-stuffed tomatoes
- wiki (fast) rice
- orange couscous with almonds, raisins, and mint

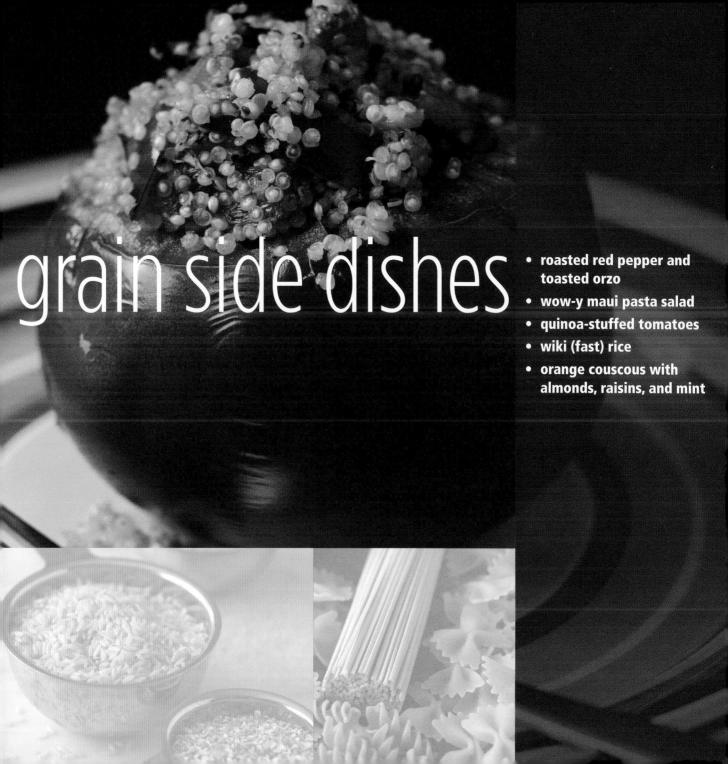

roasted red pepper and toasted orzo

pair this rich side dish with grilled chicken or fish

1 C	dry whole-grain orzo (pasta)
1 Tbsp	olive oil
1 tsp	garlic, minced (about 1 clove)
1 C	jarred roasted red peppers in natural juice, drained and diced *(or substitute fresh roasted red peppers; see tip) (Leftover Friendly)*
2 C	low-sodium chicken broth
1 Tbsp	fresh basil, rinsed, dried, and chopped (or 1 tsp dried)
1 Tbsp	fresh parsley, rinsed, dried, and chopped (or 1 tsp dried)
½ C	shredded part skim mozzarella cheese

1. Preheat oven to 400 °F. Place orzo on a baking sheet and toast in the oven for 5 minutes, or until it just begins to brown (or brown in a saucepan). Remove from heat and cool slightly.
2. Heat olive oil in a medium saucepan over medium heat. Add garlic, and cook gently until it gets soft, but does not brown (about 30 seconds).
3. Add peppers, and cook until heated through.
4. Add toasted orzo and chicken broth. Bring to a boil and simmer gently, stirring often until the pasta has absorbed all of the liquid and is fully cooked, about 10–15 minutes. (If necessary, add 2 more tablespoons broth at a time, up to ¼ cup.)
5. Add herbs and cheese. Toss gently to mix; do not overmix or the cheese will become gummy. Serve immediately.

Tip: To make roasted red peppers, see instructions in the FAQs in appendix D (on page 108). Make extra to use in other Keep the Beat™ recipes.

Substitute fresh roasted red peppers by making extra when you make the **Super Quick Chunky Tomato Sauce** (on page 54). If you don't have leftover cooked vegetables, see basic cooking instructions in appendix D (page 103).

prep time: 10 minutes	**yield:** 4 servings		
cook time: 25 minutes	**serving size:** 1 C pasta		

each serving provides:

calories	205	carbohydrates	24 g
total fat	7 g	potassium	126 mg
saturated fat	2 g	vitamin A	4%
cholesterol	9 mg	vitamin C	4%
sodium	234 mg	calcium	10%
total fiber	5 g	iron	2%
protein	9 g		

Percent Daily Values are based on a 2,000 calorie diet.

wow-y maui pasta salad

try this flavorful side dish with the **Hawaiian Huli Huli Chicken** (on page 13)—
or it's perfect for a summer party!

2 C	dry whole-wheat rotini (spiral) pasta (8 oz)
1 C	fresh or frozen snow peapods, sliced thinly on an angle (julienned)
½ C	cucumber, peeled and diced
¼ C	carrots, peeled and diced
1 can	(8 oz) pineapple chunks in juice, diced; set aside ¼ C juice
½ C	fat-free plain yogurt
1 Tbsp	fresh chives, rinsed, dried, and chopped (or 1 tsp dried)
1 Tbsp	fresh parsley, rinsed, dried, and chopped (or 1 tsp dried)
¼ tsp	salt
¼ tsp	ground black pepper

1. In a 4-quart saucepan, bring 3 quarts of water to a boil over high heat. Add pasta, and cook until tender, about 8 minutes. Drain, cool, and set aside.
2. In the meantime, place peapods in a microwavable dish, add enough water to keep moist, and microwave for 1–2 minutes, or until warm.
3. Meanwhile, combine the remaining ingredients together in a separate bowl, and toss gently.
4. Add cooked pasta and peapods, and toss gently to coat the pasta.
5. Serve immediately, or refrigerate for later use.

This is a great recipe for older children to make themselves. Younger children can help peel the cucumber and carrots.

prep time: 15 minutes	**yield:** 4 servings	
cook time: 15 minutes	**serving size:** 2 C pasta salad	

each serving provides:

calories	273	carbohydrates	56 g
total fat	2 g	potassium	207 mg
saturated fat	0 g	vitamin A	35%
cholesterol	1 mg	vitamin C	50%
sodium	171 mg	calcium	8%
total fiber	7 g	iron	6%
protein	10 g		

Percent Daily Values are based on a 2,000 calorie diet.

grain side dishes

quinoa-stuffed tomatoes

quinoa (pronounced KEEN-wah) is a grain native to South America; children will have fun eating quinoa out of a hollowed-out tomato

4	medium (2½ inches) tomatoes, rinsed
1 Tbsp	olive oil
2 Tbsp	red onions, peeled and chopped
1 C	cooked mixed vegetables—such as peppers, corn, carrots, or peas *(Leftover Friendly)*
1 C	quinoa, rinsed*
1 C	low-sodium chicken broth
½	ripe avocado, peeled and diced *(see tip)*
¼ tsp	ground black pepper
1 Tbsp	fresh parsley, rinsed, dried, and chopped (or 1 tsp dried)

1. Preheat oven to 350 °F.
2. Cut off the tops of the tomatoes and hollow out the insides. (The pulp can be saved for use in tomato soup or sauce, or salsa.) Set tomatoes aside.
3. Heat oil in a saucepan over medium-high heat. Add onions, and cook until they begin to soften, about 1–2 minutes.
4. Add cooked vegetables, and heat through, about another 1–2 minutes.

continued on page 59

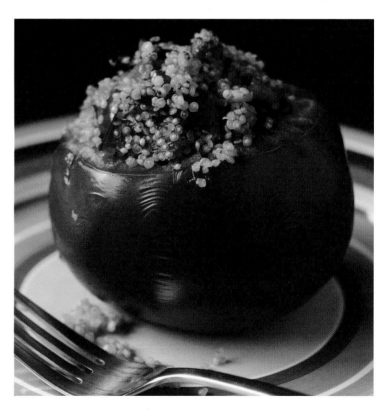

quinoa-stuffed tomatoes (continued)

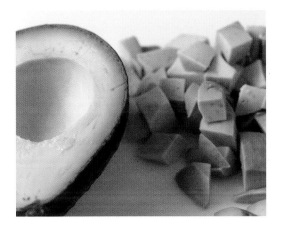

5. Add quinoa, and cook gently until it smells good, about 2 minutes.

6. Add chicken broth, and bring to a boil. Reduce the heat and cover the pan. Cook until the quinoa has absorbed all of the liquid and is fully cooked, about 7–10 minutes.

7. When the quinoa is cooked, remove the lid and gently fluff quinoa with a fork. Gently mix in the avocado, pepper, and parsley.

8. Carefully stuff about ¾ cup of quinoa into each tomato.

9. Place tomatoes on a baking sheet, and bake for about 15–20 minutes, or until tomatoes are hot throughout (tomatoes may be stuffed in advance and baked later).

10. Serve immediately.

Tip: See appendix D for a description of how to choose, peel, and cut an avocado. Use the other half of the avocado for the **Tuna and Avocado Cobb Salad** (on page 37).

* Unprocessed quinoa must be washed thoroughly before it is used to remove a powdery coating called saponin, which has an unpleasant and bitter taste. Check your package for rinsing instructions.

If you don't have leftover cooked vegetables, see basic cooking instructions in appendix D (page 103).

prep time:	yield:	each serving provides:			
10 minutes	4 servings	calories	299	carbohydrates	46 g
		total fat	10 g	potassium	906 mg
cook time:	serving size:	saturated fat	1 g	vitamin A	110%
35–40 minutes	1 tomato,	cholesterol	0 mg	vitamin C	40%
	¾ C stuffing	sodium	64 mg	calcium	6%
		total fiber	8 g	iron	30%
		protein	10 g		

Percent Daily Values are based on a 2,000 calorie diet.

grain side dishes

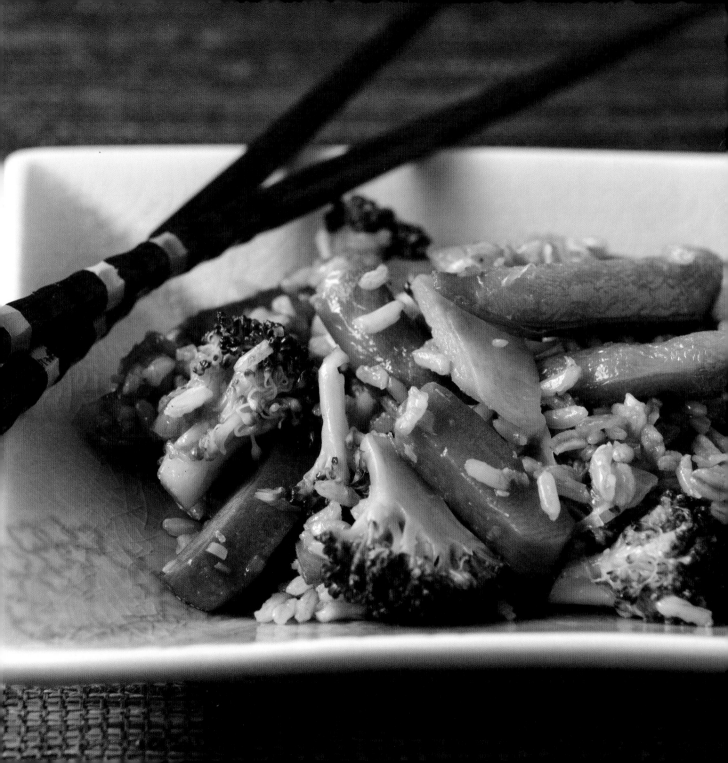

wiki (fast) rice

wiki means "fast" in Hawaiian, and this dish fits the bill—it's quick and easy to make

1 Tbsp	canola oil
1 Tbsp	fresh garlic, minced (about 3 cloves) (or 1 tsp dried)
1 tsp	fresh ginger, minced (or ¼ tsp dried)
1 Tbsp	scallions (green onions), rinsed and minced
½ C	canned sliced water chestnuts, drained
2 C	cooked mixed vegetables (or ½ bag frozen stir-fry vegetable mix) *(Leftover Friendly)*
2 C	cooked brown rice *(Leftover Friendly)*
1 Tbsp	lite soy sauce
1 tsp	sesame oil

1. Heat canola oil in a large wok or sauté pan over medium heat. Add garlic, ginger, and scallions, and cook until fragrant, about 1 minute.
2. Add water chestnuts, and continue to cook until they begin to soften, another 1–2 minutes.
3. Add vegetables, and toss until heated through, about 2–3 minutes (or up to 5 minutes for frozen vegetables).
4. Add rice, and continue to cook until hot, about 3–5 minutes.
5. Add soy sauce and sesame oil. Toss well, and serve.

This recipe tastes best when prepared using leftover cold rice. If you don't have leftover cooked vegetables, see basic cooking instructions in appendix D (page 103).

prep time:
10 minutes

cook time:
15 minutes

yield:
4 servings

serving size:
about 1 C rice and vegetables

each serving provides:

calories	179	carbohydrates	29 g
total fat	6 g	potassium	88 mg
saturated fat	1 g	vitamin A	4%
cholesterol	0 mg	vitamin C	15%
sodium	113 mg	calcium	2%
total fiber	2 g	iron	4%
protein	4 g		

Percent Daily Values are based on a 2,000 calorie diet.

grain side dishes

orange couscous with almonds, raisins, and mint

this flavorful side dish goes well with chicken, beef, or lamb

1¼ C	low-sodium chicken broth
2 Tbsp	raisins
1 C	whole-wheat couscous
1 Tbsp	fresh mint, rinsed, dried, and chopped (or 1 tsp dried)
1 Tbsp	unsalted sliced almonds, toasted
1	medium orange, rinsed, for 1 Tbsp zest (*use a grater to take a thin layer of skin off the orange*)

1. Combine chicken broth and raisins in a small saucepan. Bring to a boil over high heat.

2. Add couscous, and return to a boil. Cover and remove from the heat.

3. Let the saucepan stand for about 5 minutes, until the couscous has absorbed all of the broth.

4. Meanwhile, toast almonds in the toaster oven on a foil-lined tray for about 5 minutes, or until golden brown.

5. Remove the lid and fluff the couscous with a fork. Gently mix in the mint, almonds, and orange zest. Serve immediately.

CHEFS IN TRAINING

This is a great recipe for older children to make themselves. Younger children can help measure ingredients and zest the orange.

prep time:	**yield:**	**each serving provides:**			
10 minutes	4 servings	calories	141	carbohydrates	28 g
		total fat	2 g	potassium	118 mg
cook time:	**serving size:**	saturated fat	0 g	vitamin A	0%
20 minutes (including 10 minutes standing time)	¾ C couscous	cholesterol	0 mg	vitamin C	4%
		sodium	24 mg	calcium	2%
		total fiber	4 g	iron	6%
		protein	6 g		

Percent Daily Values are based on a 2,000 calorie diet.

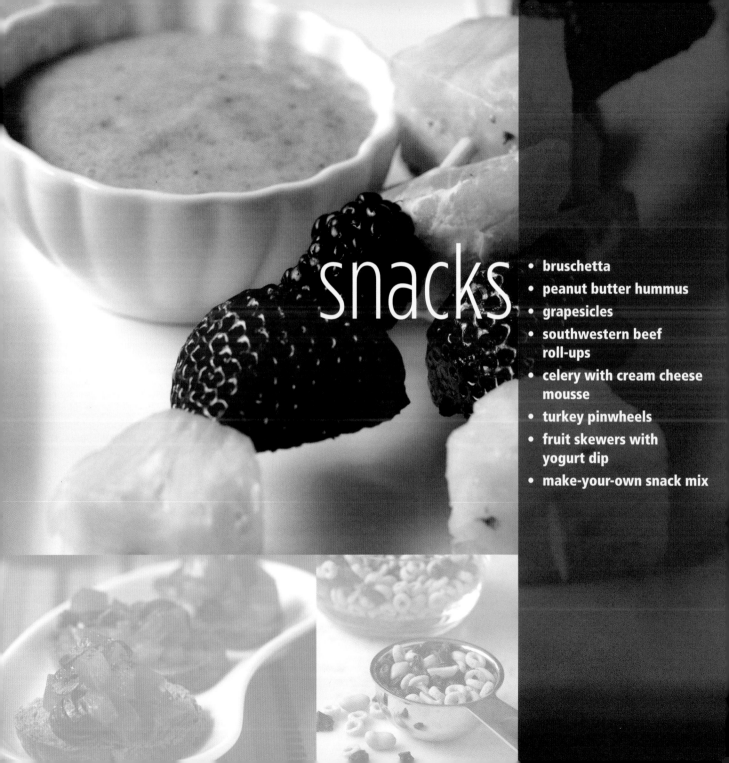

snacks

- **bruschetta**
- **peanut butter hummus**
- **grapesicles**
- **southwestern beef roll-ups**
- **celery with cream cheese mousse**
- **turkey pinwheels**
- **fruit skewers with yogurt dip**
- **make-your-own snack mix**

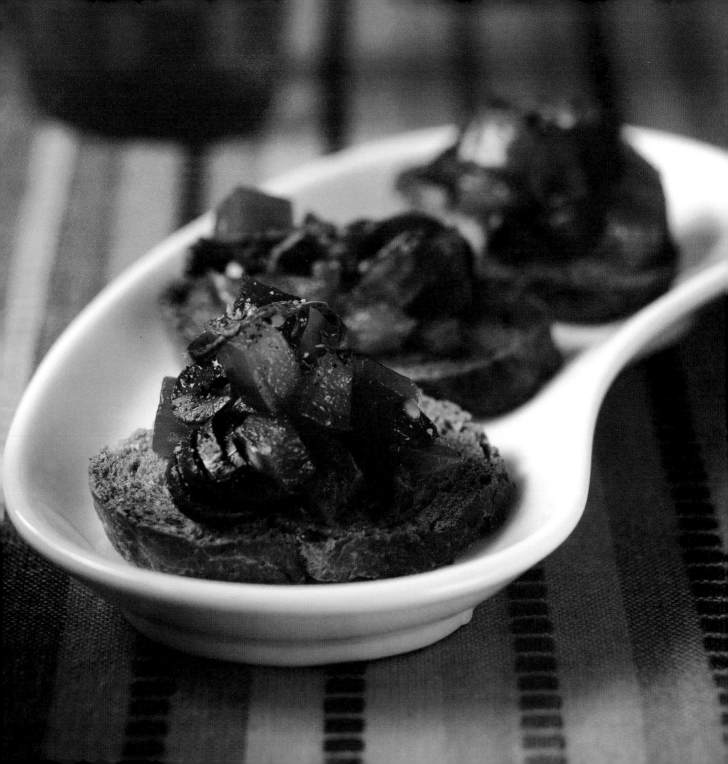

bruschetta

roasted red peppers add extra zing to this classic chopped tomato dish

½	whole grain baguette (French bread), cut into 12 slices *(or substitute 3 slices whole-wheat bread, each cut into 4 squares)*
1 C	fresh tomatoes, rinsed and diced
¼ C	jarred roasted red peppers, diced *(or substitute fresh roasted red peppers; see tip) (Leftover Friendly)*
6	Kalamata olives, rinsed and sliced *(or substitute any black olive)*
½ Tbsp	olive oil
2 Tbsp	fresh basil, rinsed, dried, and chopped (or 2 tsp dried)
¼ tsp	ground black pepper

1. Lightly toast baguette slices.
2. Combine remaining ingredients, and toss well.
3. Top each bread slice with about 2 tablespoons of tomato mixture, and serve.

Tip: To make roasted red peppers, see instructions in the FAQs in appendix D (on page 108). Make extra to use in other Keep the Beat™ recipes.

 Substitute fresh roasted red peppers by making extra when you make the **Super Quick Chunky Tomato Sauce** (on page 54). If you don't have leftover cooked vegetables, see basic cooking instructions in appendix D (page 103).

 Younger children can help arrange the sliced bread on the tray and add the toppings. Older children can make the recipe themselves.

prep time: 15 minutes	**yield:** 4 servings		
cook time: 5 minutes	**serving size:** 3 bruschetta slices, each with 2 Tbsp tomato mixture		

each serving provides:

calories	119	carbohydrates	17 g
total fat	4 g	potassium	113 mg
saturated fat	0 g	vitamin A	10%
cholesterol	0 mg	vitamin C	10%
sodium	256 mg	calcium	4%
total fiber	2 g	iron	6%
protein	4 g		

Percent Daily Values are based on a 2,000 calorie diet.

peanut butter hummus

bring out the veggies or pita chips—try this irresistible combination of peanut butter and hummus . . . with a spicy kick!

For dip:

2 C	low-sodium garbanzo beans (chick peas), rinsed
¼ C	low-sodium chicken broth
¼ C	lemon juice
2–3 Tbsp	garlic, diced (about 4–6 garlic cloves, depending on taste)
¼ C	creamy peanut butter *(or substitute other nut or seed butter)*
¼ tsp	cayenne pepper *(or substitute paprika for less spice)*
1 Tbsp	olive oil

For pita chips:

4	(6½-inch) whole-wheat pitas, each cut into 10 triangles
1 Tbsp	olive oil
1 tsp	garlic, minced (about 1 clove) (or ½ tsp garlic powder)
¼ tsp	ground black pepper

1. Preheat oven to 400 °F.
2. To prepare the hummus, combine all ingredients for the dip and mix them in a food processor or blender. Puree until smooth.
3. To prepare the chips, toss the pita triangles with the olive oil, garlic, and pepper.
4. Bake chips on a baking sheet in a 400 °F oven for 10 minutes, or until crispy.
5. Arrange pita chips on a platter, and serve with the hummus.

Note: If you can't find beans that are labeled "low sodium," compare the Nutrition Facts panels to find the beans with the lowest amount of sodium. Rinsing can help reduce sodium levels further.

Younger children can break apart the pita bread. Older children can make the recipe themselves.

prep time: 20 minutes	**yield:** 8 servings	**each serving provides:**	
		calories	235
		total fat	9 g
cook time: 10 minutes	**serving size:** ⅓ C hummus and 5 pita chips	saturated fat	1 g
		cholesterol	0 mg
		sodium	225 mg
		total fiber	5 g
		protein	9 g

carbohydrates	32 g
potassium	259 mg
vitamin A	0%
vitamin C	8%
calcium	4%
iron	10%

Percent Daily Values are based on a 2,000 calorie diet.

grapesicles

try this healthy snack on a hot summer day—frozen grapes will pop in your mouth!

48	green seedless grapes, rinsed
48	red seedless grapes, rinsed
16	6-inch wooden skewers

1. Thread six grapes, alternating grape colors, onto each wooden skewer.
2. Place skewers into the freezer for 30 minutes, or until frozen.
3. Serve immediately.

Note: Skewers have sharp edges, so monitor younger children while eating, or take the grapes off the skewers for them. Grapes should be cut in half for children under 3 years old to prevent choking.

CHEFS IN TRAINING

Children can rinse the grapes, freeze them, and thread the skewers.

prep time:
5 minutes

freeze time:
30 minutes

yield:
4 servings

serving size:
4 skewers

each serving provides:

calories	83	carbohydrates	22 g
total fat	0 g	potassium	229 mg
saturated fat	0 g	vitamin A	2%
cholesterol	0 mg	vitamin C	20%
sodium	2 mg	calcium	2%
total fiber	1 g	iron	6%
protein	1 g		

Percent Daily Values are based on a 2,000 calorie diet.

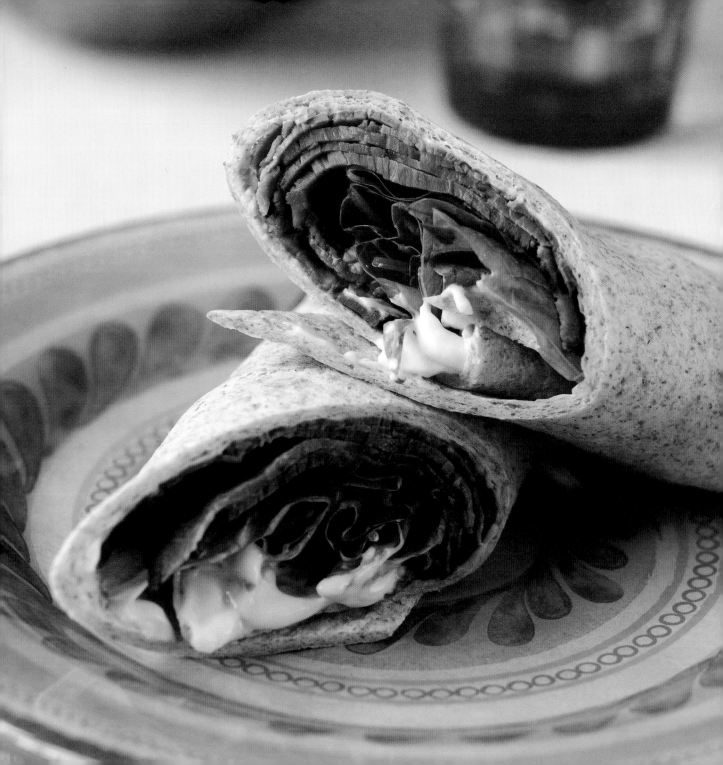

southwestern beef roll-ups

this tasty snack is simple to make and a good source of protein

4	whole-wheat tortillas (6½ inch)
4	red leaf lettuce leaves, rinsed and dried
4 oz	low-sodium deli roast beef

For spread:

1 Tbsp	light mayonnaise
1 tsp	lime juice (about ½ fresh lime)
½ tsp	hot sauce

1. Combine ingredients for the spread. Mix well.
2. Spread about 1 teaspoon of spread on each tortilla.
3. Top each tortilla with one lettuce leaf and 1 ounce roast beef (about two slices).
4. Fold sides in, and roll.
5. Serve with a side of **Tangy Salsa** (on page 51).

Younger children can mix the spread. Older children can prepare the recipe themselves.

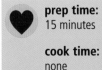

prep time:	yield:	each serving provides:			
15 minutes	4 servings	calories	190	carbohydrates	23 g
		total fat	5 g	potassium	36 mg
cook time:	**serving size:**	saturated fat	0 g	vitamin A	25%
none	1 tortilla	cholesterol	21 mg	vitamin C	2%
		sodium	302 mg	calcium	4%
		total fiber	2 g	iron	7%
		protein	11 g		

Percent Daily Values are based on a 2,000 calorie diet.

celery with cream cheese mousse

this delicious and light snack will please the young . . . and young at heart

¼ C	low-fat whipped cream cheese
¼ C	fat-free plain yogurt
2 Tbsp	scallions (green onions), rinsed and chopped
1 Tbsp	lemon juice
½ tsp	ground black pepper
6	celery sticks, rinsed, with ends cut off
1 Tbsp	chopped walnuts

1. Combine cream cheese, yogurt, scallions, lemon juice, and pepper. Mix well with a wooden spoon.

2. Spread mixture evenly down the middle of each celery stick.

3. Cut each stick into 5 pieces. Top with chopped walnuts, and serve.

Younger children can help mix the "mousse." Older children can make the recipe themselves.

prep time:
10 minutes

cook time:
none

yield:
6 servings

serving size:
2 Tbsp of mousse
with 1 celery stick
(5 pieces)

each serving provides:

calories	35	carbohydrates	3 g
total fat	2 g	potassium	131 mg
saturated fat	1 g	vitamin A	6%
cholesterol	4 mg	vitamin C	6%
sodium	58 mg	calcium	4%
total fiber	1 g	iron	2%
protein	2 g		

Percent Daily Values are based on a 2,000 calorie diet.

turkey pinwheels
this fun-to-make snack will become a family favorite

4 slices	whole-wheat bread
1 Tbsp	light mayonnaise
1 Tbsp	deli mustard
½ C	cucumber, peeled and thinly sliced
¼ C	jarred roasted red peppers
2 oz	low-sodium deli turkey breast

1. Remove the crusts from the bread and flatten each slice with a rolling pin.
2. Combine mayonnaise and mustard. Spread about ½ tablespoon on each bread slice.
3. Arrange cucumbers and red peppers evenly on each slice of bread, and top with ½ ounce turkey.
4. Roll each slice into a log, and cut each log into four pieces with a sharp knife. Serve immediately, or refrigerate logs until ready to serve (cut prior to serving).

Younger children can help flatten the bread and roll the logs. Older children can make the recipe themselves.

prep time:
10 minutes

cook time:
none

yield:
4 servings

serving size:
1 log (4 pieces)

each serving provides:

calories	106	carbohydrates	12 g
total fat	2 g	potassium	25 mg
saturated fat	0 g	vitamin A	0%
cholesterol	11 mg	vitamin C	0%
sodium	275 mg	calcium	2%
total fiber	2 g	iron	4%
protein	7 g		

Percent Daily Values are based on a 2,000 calorie diet.

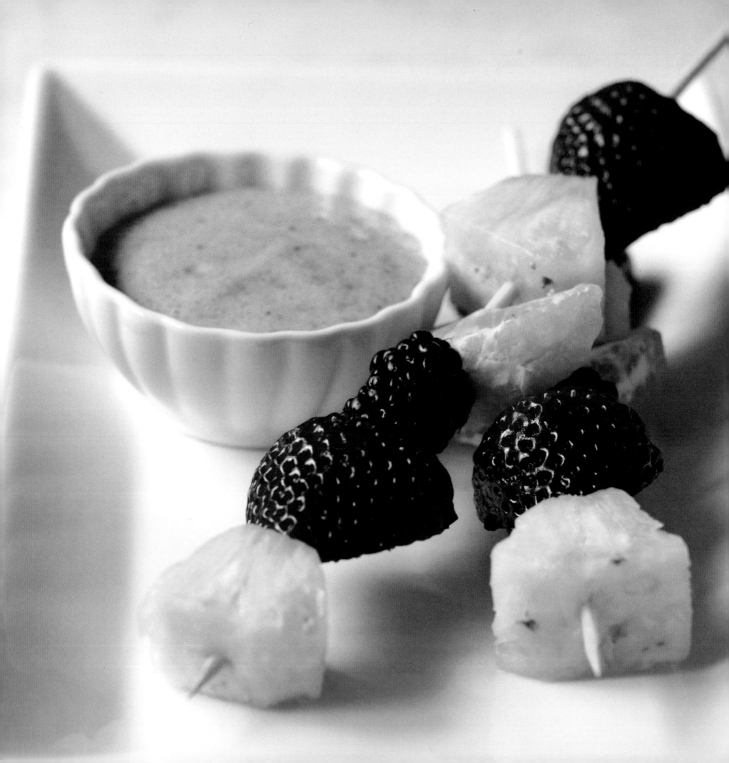

fruit skewers with yogurt dip

tangy fruit and sweet yogurt make a perfect taste combination

1 C strawberries, rinsed, stems removed, and cut in half

1 C fresh pineapple, diced (or canned pineapple chunks in juice, drained)

½ C blackberries

1 tangerine or Clementine, peeled and cut into 8 segments

8 6-inch wooden skewers

For dip:

1 C strawberries, rinsed, stems removed, and cut in half

¼ C fat-free plain yogurt

⅛ tsp vanilla extract

1 Tbsp honey

1. Thread two strawberry halves, two pineapple chunks, two blackberries, and one tangerine segment on each skewer.

2. To prepare the dip, puree strawberries in a blender or food processor. Add yogurt, vanilla, and honey, and mix well.

3. Serve two skewers with yogurt dip on the side.

Note: Skewers have sharp edges, so monitor younger children while eating, or take the fruit off the skewers for them.

Younger children can rinse the fruit, thread onto skewers, and mix the dip. Older children can make the recipe themselves.

prep time: 15 minutes	**yield:** 4 servings	**each serving provides:**			
		calories	71	carbohydrates	18 g
cook time: none	**serving size:** 2 skewers, 1½ Tbsp dip	total fat	0 g	potassium	174 mg
		saturated fat	0 g	vitamin A	6%
		cholesterol	0 mg	vitamin C	70%
		sodium	10 mg	calcium	4%
		total fiber	2 g	iron	2%
		protein	1 g		

Percent Daily Values are based on a 2,000 calorie diet.

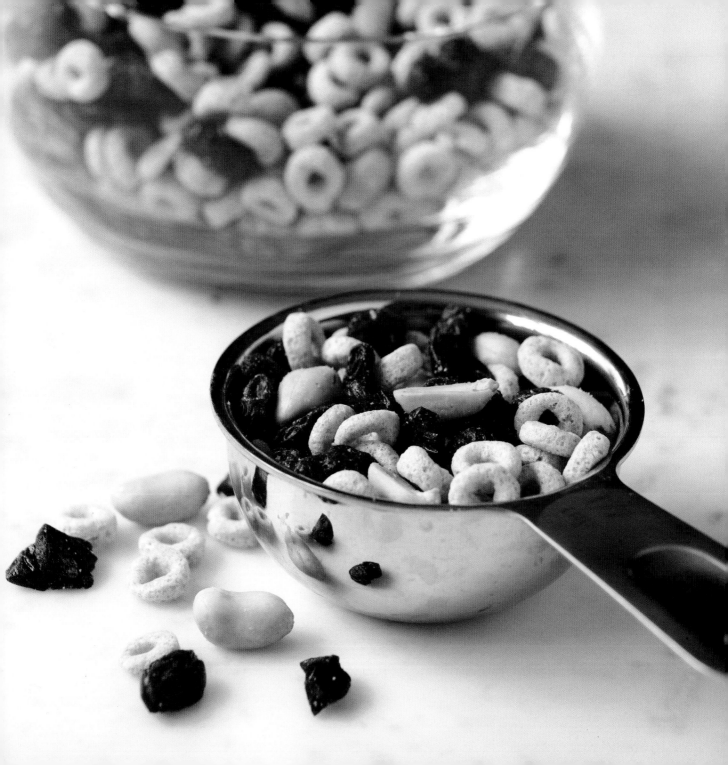

make-your-own snack mix

making your own snack mix can be healthier and less expensive than buying it

1 C	toasted oat cereal	
¼ C	unsalted dry roasted peanuts (or other unsalted nut)	
¼ C	raisins	
¼ C	dried cranberries	

1. Combine all ingredients, and toss well.
2. Serve immediately, or store for later snacking.

Tip: Put snack mix in individual snack-sized bags for a great grab-and-go snack.

Most children can make this recipe themselves.

---

prep time: 5 minutes	**yield:** 4 servings	**each serving provides:**			
		calories	136	carbohydrates	22 g
cook time: none	**serving size:** ½ C snack mix	total fat	5 g	potassium	170 mg
		saturated fat	1 g	vitamin A	4%
		cholesterol	0 mg	vitamin C	4%
		sodium	75 mg	calcium	2%
		total fiber	2 g	iron	15%
		protein	3 g		

Percent Daily Values are based on a 2,000 calorie diet.

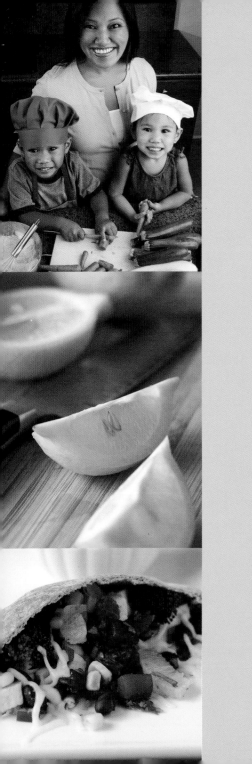

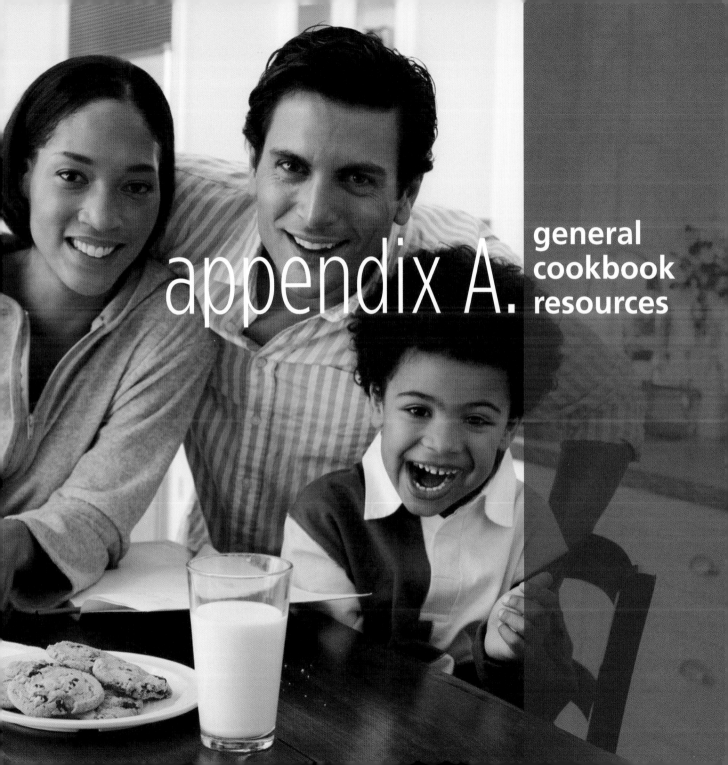

appendix A. general cookbook resources

about *We Can!* ®

Keep the Beat™ Recipes: Deliciously Healthy Family Meals was developed in collaboration with the National Institutes of Health (NIH) *We Can!*® program.

We Can! (**W**ays to **E**nhance **C**hildren's **A**ctivity & **N**utrition) is a national education program designed to give parents, caregivers, and entire communities a way to help children stay at a healthy weight.

Four NIH Institutes have come together to bring you *We Can!*, including the NHLBI, the National Institute of Diabetes and Digestive and Kidney Diseases, the *Eunice Kennedy Shriver* National Institute of Child Health and Human Development, and the National Cancer Institute. These Institutes have combined their unique resources and activities to make *We Can!* a national success.

for parents, families, and caregivers

Research shows that parents and caregivers are a primary influencer of children. The *We Can!* program provides parents and caregivers with tips, tools, fun activities, and more to help them encourage healthy eating, increase their family's physical activity, and reduce the time family members spend sitting in front of the screen (TV or computer). Learn more about healthy weight basics and how to help your family make healthy lifestyle choices by exploring the appendixes in this recipe book and by visiting the *We Can!* Web site.

for partners

We Can! also offers organizations, community groups, and health professionals a centralized resource to promote a healthy weight in youth through community outreach, partnership development, and media activities that can be adapted to meet the needs of diverse populations. Science-based educational programs, support materials, training opportunities, and other resources are available to support programming for youth, parents, and communities.

A growing number of organizations are helping spread *We Can!* programming from coast to coast, from North to South, and to various points around the world. These include communities, corporations, national organizations, and professional societies across the Nation that are playing an active role in creating healthier hometowns with *We Can!*. Visit the Web site to find out how to partner with the program.

for health professionals

Many families look to their family physicians, pediatricians, or other health care professionals for instructions on how to help their children adopt healthier habits. Visit the For Health Professionals section of the *We Can!* Web site to find practical tips about healthier lifestyles.

for more information

For more information about *We Can!*, go to http://wecan.nhlbi.nih.gov.

guide to recipe symbols

healthier classics symbol

Classic favorites that are made healthier by reducing fat, calories, and/or sodium. Healthier classics also could have more vegetables or whole grains added than original versions.

leftover friendly symbol

Recipes that use leftover ingredients to help save cooking time.

chefs in training symbol

Tips for getting children involved in meal preparation.

healthy eating two ways symbol

Simple tips to serve a recipe two ways to please picky eaters and other family members.

side dish recommendations

- With the Emapañapita (page 7)—try a side of Tangy Salsa ....page 51
- With the Baked Eggrolls (page 11)—try a side of Wiki (Fast) Rice..........page 61
- With the Hawaiian Huli Huli Chicken (page 13)—try a side of
  Wow-y Maui Pasta Salad..page 57
- With the Turkey and Beef Meatballs With Whole-Wheat Spaghetti
  (page 25)—try a side of Parmesan Green Beans ....page 52
- Use the Super Quick Chunky Tomato Sauce (page 54) in these dishes:
  - Mexican Lasagna..page 19
  - Turkey and Beef Meatballs With Whole-Wheat Spaghetti ....page 25
  - Pita Pizzas ....page 35

appendix A

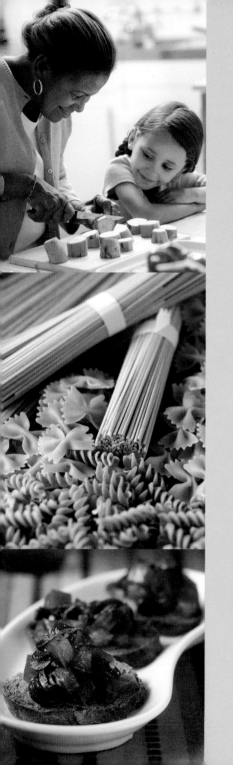

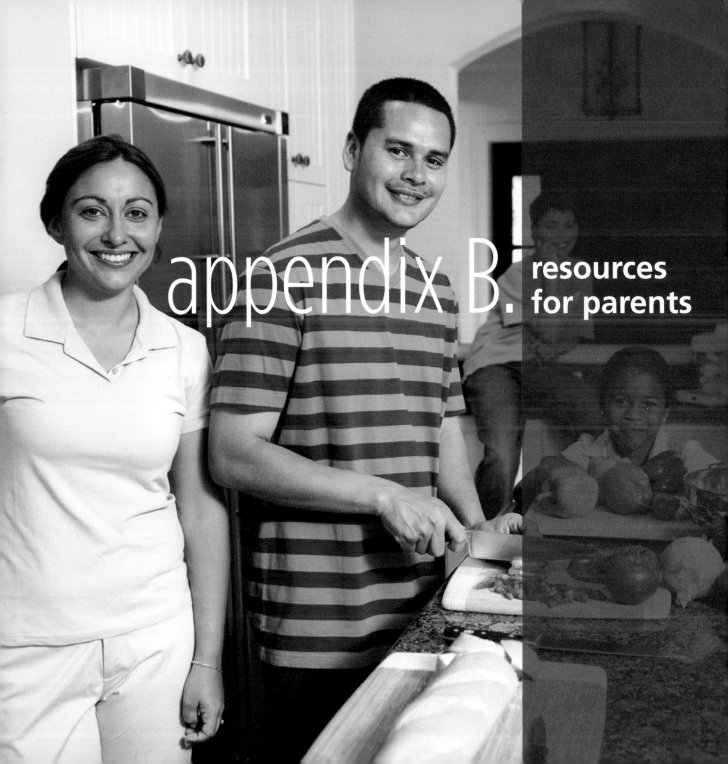

appendix B. **resources for parents**

what can my family and I do to encourage a healthy weight?

You may be asking what you can do in your own family to prevent overweight and obesity. The two main ways to encourage and maintain a healthy weight are to make smart food choices and to be physically active.

As parents, you make a big difference in what your children think and do. If you eat right and are physically active, there's a good chance your children will be too. Together, families can be more successful in adopting healthy choices and making changes. Creating family habits around smart eating and physical activity can make it easier for everyone to maintain a healthy weight. For example:

- Planning regular family time that involves physical activity means that everyone is supported and encouraged to be active.

- Putting a bowl of fruit on the kitchen counter and making a family agreement not to have chips or other high-calorie snacks in the house can change everyone's snacking habits.

strategies for real life

If you're interested in jump-starting your family on a healthy lifestyle by making some nutrition and physical activity changes, here are a few strategies to get you started:

- **Recognize that you have more control than you might think.** *You* can turn off the TV and video games. *You* can park your car farther away from the store. *You* can give your family more vegetables with dinner.

- **Think about immediate benefits.** If reducing future heart disease risk seems a bit abstract, focus on the good things that can happen right now. You won't feel so full if you have a smaller portion of dessert, or have a piece of fruit instead. Going hiking with your teenager might lead to a wonderful talk that neither of you anticipated. A vegetable salad tastes great and looks beautiful. Dancing with your spouse is lots of fun and can give you a great workout.

- **Make small changes over time.** It's easier and more appealing to start out with some new approaches to nutrition and physical activity that the whole family is willing to try. For example, shoot some baskets after dinner a few nights a week instead of turning on the TV. Start your weekend by taking a walk with your family or a trip to a local farmer's market. And, instead of chocolate cake with frosting, enjoy sliced strawberries over angel food cake.

- **Try a variety of strategies.** No one will notice if you use part-skim mozzarella cheese instead of whole-milk mozzarella in your lasagna, but you'll be reducing the number of calories and fat for everyone who eats it. Combine "invisible" strategies like this with strategies that actively involve other family members: See whether everyone will commit to eating healthy dinners at least four times a week. Get your children involved in the process of shopping for and preparing these healthy dinners. Make a plan with your child to walk to school together or to walk after dinner 2 days a week.

For more information and tips on eating healthier at home, read *We Can! Families Finding the Balance: A Parent Handbook* (available online at http://wecan.nhlbi.nih.gov).

time-saving tips for busy families

Like most families, your life is probably busy with work, school, activities, and other commitments, and you may feel like you don't have enough time to put healthy food on the table. However, cooking healthy meals for your family can be simple and delicious with easy recipes and a little advance planning. Here are some tips to make healthy cooking at home easier.

menu planning and shopping

- **Make a plan and stick to it.** Choose one day each week to plan meals for the week. Then create a grocery list based on your meal plan. A little planning ahead can help save you lots of time and money. Try using these tools on the *We Can!* Web site (http://wecan.nhlbi.nih.gov):

  - *We Can!* Weekly Meal Planner

  - *We Can!* Grocery Shopping List Template

- **Make planning a family affair.** Ask your family to help you write the weekly meal plan and grocery list—post these materials on the refrigerator and ask family members to help fill them out as they come up with ideas.

- **Plan for leftovers and "batch" cooking when making your grocery list.** For example, if you know you won't have leftover Hawaiian Huli Huli Chicken (page 13), then plan to make extra chicken and sauce for an easy meal of "Fried" Rice and Chicken (page 15). Or, roast several red peppers at once to batch cook for the Tangy Salsa (page 51), Super Quick Chunky Tomato Sauce (page 54), and Roasted Red Pepper and Toasted Orzo (page 56).

- **Stock your kitchen** with staple healthy ingredients such as brown rice, whole-wheat pasta, sundried tomatoes, frozen shrimp, chicken breast, canned low-sodium beans, no-salt-added diced tomatoes, frozen vegetables with no added sauce, etc. For more healthy ingredient ideas, visit the Keep the Beat™: Deliciously Healthy Eating Web site (http://hin.nhlbi.nih.gov/healthyeating).

- **Shop smart.** Stick to your grocery list to avoid buying items you don't need. Time your grocery trip for when the store is less crowded and you're not rushed or hungry. Get the recipe ingredients and other foods on your list in just one trip.

preparation

- Read over each recipe before starting so you know what's involved. Lay out all of the ingredients and tools you'll need (measuring cups, spoons, knives, cutting board, pots and pans, etc.) to get organized before cooking.

- Chop all ingredients before you start cooking.

- Carefully plan when to start preparing side dishes so everything is ready at once.

- Ask your children to help set the table and even help prepare dishes. (In recipes in this cookbook, the Chefs in Training symbol identifies tips on how to get children involved in food preparation.)

cooking

- Use quick recipes with few ingredients (such as the ones in this cookbook).

- Cook once, eat twice. (See Menu Planning and Shopping and Storing sections for more information. Also, in this cookbook, the Leftover Friendly symbol identifies ingredients that you might have as leftovers from previous meals.)

storing

- Store leftover meals in the refrigerator for lunch the next day, or freeze for a later time.

- Refrigerate or freeze leftover cooked ingredients (veggies, chicken, rice, etc.) so they're ready to quickly toss into recipes another time.

- For information on storing food safely, refer to:

  - The Federal Food Safety Web site at www.foodsafety.gov.

  - The USDA Food Safety and Inspection Service's Meat and Poultry Hotline: 1–888–674–6854.

for more tips and tools

See the Keep the Beat™: Deliciously Healthy Eating Web site (http://hin.nhlbi.nih. gov/healthyeating) for more tips and tools for healthy cooking.

We Can! parent tips: making healthier food choices

As a parent, you want to give your family the best food you can. Serving healthier foods in the appropriate servings per food group and calorie level is one of the best ways to ensure that your children are getting proper nutrition without eating too many calories. The simple tips provided here and on the *We Can!* Web site (http://wecan.nhlbi.nih.gov) can help you plan and prepare meals and snacks to help your family get the most out of the calories they consume.

what is a "healthy" diet?

The U.S. Dietary Guidelines for Americans describes a healthy eating plan as one that:

- Emphasizes fruits, vegetables, whole grains, and fat-free or low-fat milk and milk products

- Includes lean meats, poultry, fish, beans, eggs, and nuts

- Is low in saturated fats, *trans* fats, cholesterol, sodium (salt), and added sugars

- Stays within your calorie needs

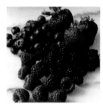 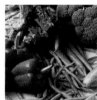 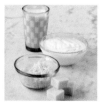 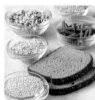 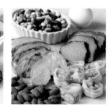

Focus on Food Choices

GO foods are the lowest in fat and added sugar. They also are "nutrient dense" (which means they are a much better source of vitamins, minerals, and other nutrients important to health) and relatively low in calories. Enjoy GO foods almost any time. Examples of GO foods are fruits (fresh, frozen, or canned in juice), vegetables (fresh, frozen without added fat, canned without added sodium), whole grains, fat-free or low-fat milk products, lean meat, poultry, fish, beans, egg whites, or egg substitute.

SLOW foods are higher in fat, added sugar, and/or calories than GO foods. SLOW foods include vegetables with added fat, white refined bread flour, low-fat mayonnaise, and 2 percent low-fat milk. Have SLOW foods sometimes or less often.

WHOA foods are the highest in fat and/or added sugar. They are "calorie dense" (which means a small portion is relatively high in calories) and may be low in vitamins, minerals, and other nutrients as well. Have WHOA foods only once in a while or on special occasions. And, when you do have them, have small portions. Examples of WHOA foods are whole milk, cheese, fried potatoes, croissants, muffins, butter, and creamy salad dressing.

To download a GO, SLOW, and WHOA Food Chart, go to the *We Can!* Web site at http://wecan.nhlbi.nih.gov.

how much should I feed my child?

Although the recipes in this cookbook were created to appeal to both adults and children, depending on their age and activity level, children may need to eat smaller servings of food than do adults. In general, children need to consume a sufficient number of calories and nutrients to promote growth; additional calories may contribute to excess weight gain.

Here are some guidelines on how much to serve children at different ages. For more information on tips for feeding children, see the Keep the Beat™: Deliciously Healthy Eating Web site (http://hin.nhlbi.nih.gov/healthyeating) and the U.S. Department of Agriculture's MyPyramid Web site (www.MyPyramid.gov).

estimated calorie requirements
in Kilocalories for each gender and age group at three levels of physical activity[a]

Gender	Age (years)	Activity Level [b,c,d]		
		Sedentary[b]	Moderately Active[c]	Active[d]
Child	2–3	1,000	1,000–1,400[e]	1,000–1,400[e]
Female	4–8	1,200	1,400–1,600	1,400–1,800
	9–13	1,600	1,600–2,000	1,800–2,200
	14–18	1,800	2,000	2,400
	19–30	2,000	2,000–2,200	2,400
	31–50	1,800	2,000	2,200
	51+	1,600	1,800	2,000–2,200
Male	4–8	1,400	1,400–1,600	1,600–2,000
	9–13	1,800	1,800–2,200	2,000–2,600
	14–18	2,200	2,400–2,800	2,800–3,200
	19–30	2,400	2,600–2,800	3,000
	31–50	2,200	2,400–2,600	2,800–3,000
	51+	2,000	2,200–2,400	2,400–2,800

Source: Dietary Guidelines for Americans, 2005

[a] These levels are based on Estimated Energy Requirements (EER) from the Institute of Medicine Dietary Reference Intakes macronutrients report, 2002, calculated by gender, age, and activity level for reference-sized individuals. "Reference size," as determined by IOM, is based on median height and weight for ages up to 18 years of age and median height and weight for that height to give a BMI of 21.5 for adult females and 22.5 for adult males.

[b] Sedentary means a lifestyle that includes only the light physical activity associated with typical day-to-day life.

[c] Moderately active means a lifestyle that includes physical activity equivalent to walking about 1.5 to 3 miles per day at 3 to 4 miles per hour, in addition to the light physical activity associated with typical day-to-day life.

[d] Active means a lifestyle that includes physical activity equivalent to walking more than 3 miles per day at 3 to 4 miles per hour, in addition to the light physical activity associated with typical day-to-day life.

[e] The calorie ranges shown are to accommodate needs of different ages within the group. For children and adolescents, more calories are needed at older ages. For adults, fewer calories are needed at older ages.

chefs in training: getting children involved in the kitchen

There are different ways to engage children in the kitchen, depending on their age and skill level. All children can help with menu planning and grocery shopping. Younger children can assist with a variety of simple tasks, from setting the table to mixing ingredients. Older children can prepare simple snacks and dishes themselves. No matter what age your children are, working with them in the kitchen can motivate them to try new and healthier foods.

tips for involving younger children

Invite your child to:

- Pick out at least one new fruit or vegetable to try, when shopping.

- Wash fruits and vegetables (try the Dunkin' Veggies and Dips on page 44).

- Rinse canned beans (try the Peanut Butter Hummus on page 66).

- Measure dried pasta, beans, vegetables, etc. (try the Buttons and Bows Pasta on page 23).

- Add premeasured ingredients to recipes (try the Make-Your-Own Snack Mix on page 75).

- Stir ingredients (try the Fruit Skewers With Yogurt Dip on page 73).

- Mash potatoes with a masher (try the Shepherd's Pie on page 8).

- Stuff ingredients into a pita pocket (try the Empañapita on page 7).

- Assemble food (try the Bruschetta on page 65 or Quinoa-Stuffed Tomatoes on page 58).

- Crumble cheese (try the Bowtie Pasta With Chicken, Broccoli, and Feta on page 27).

tips for involving older children

Invite your child to:

- Peel and slice carrots, cucumbers, potatoes, etc. (try the Wow-y Maui Pasta Salad on page 57).

- Pour batter onto the griddle (try the Oatmeal Pecan Waffles (or Pancakes) on page 39).

- Flip pancakes (try the Spinach and Corn Pancakes on page 53).

- Form meatballs (try the Turkey and Beef Meatballs With Whole-Wheat Spaghetti on page 25).

- Coat chicken strips in egg and cereal batter (try the Crunchy Chicken Fingers With Tangy Dipping Sauce on page 3).

- Clean countertop surfaces and utensils.

- Slice tomatoes (try the Watermelon and Tomato Salad on page 43).

- Thread food onto skewers (try the Grapesicles on page 67).

- Help make fresh-roasted red peppers (used in multiple recipes in this cookbook).

- Make a side dish (try the Broccoli and Cheese on page 47).

- Make his or her own meal (try the Pita Pizzas on page 35).

Note: *It is up to parents to determine what tasks their children can handle.*

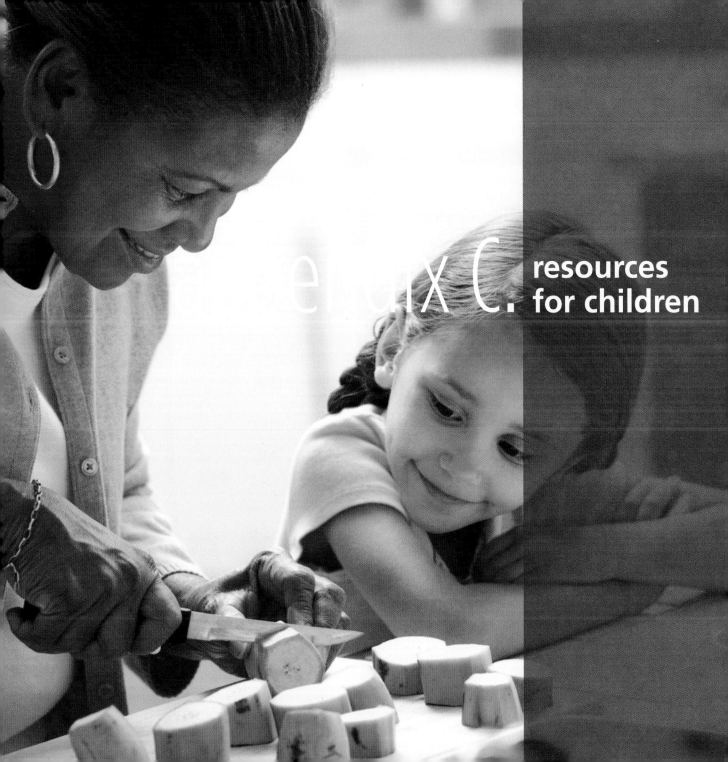

appendix C. resources
for children

a food guide for children

U R What U Eat

Food supplies the nutrients needed to fuel your body so you can perform your best. Go, Slow, Whoa is a simple way to recognize foods that are the smartest choices.
- **"Go"** Foods: Eat almost anytime (Most often) — they are lowest in fat, added sugar, and calories
- **"Slow"** Foods: Eat sometimes (Less often) — they are higher in fat, added sugar, and/or calories
- **"Whoa"** Foods: Eat once in a while (Least often) — they are very high in fat and/or added sugar, and are much higher in calories

Food Groups	GO	SLOW	WHOA
Fruits Whole fruits (fresh, frozen, canned, dried) are smart choices. You need **2 cups** of fruit a day. 1 cup is about the size of a baseball.			
Vegetables Adding fat (butter, oils, and sauces) to vegetables turns them from Go foods to Slow or Whoa foods. You need **2 ½ cups** of vegetables a day. Dark green and orange vegetables are smart choices.			
Grains Try to make at least half of your servings whole grain choices and low in sugar. An ounce of a grain product is 1 slice of bread, 1 cup of dry cereal, or ½ cup of cooked rice or pasta. You need about **6 ounces** a day.			
Milk Milk products are high in vitamins and minerals. Fat-free and low-fat milk and milk products are smart choices. About **3 cups** are needed each day; 1 cup of milk, 1 cup of yogurt or 1 ½ ounces of natural cheese count as 1 cup.			
Meats & Beans Eating **5 ½ oz.** a day will give you the protein, vitamins and minerals you need. Limit meats with added fat. Smart choices include beans (¼ cup cooked), nuts (½ oz.) and lean meats (1 oz.) baked or broiled.			

The amounts of foods recommended per food group are based on a 2,000-calorie diet, the approximate number of calories for most active boys and girls ages 9-13. U.S. Department of Agriculture, Center for Nutrition Policy and Promotion.

Sweets and Snacks

The foods below are snack-type foods. The "Slow" and "Whoa" foods are higher in fat, added sugar, and/or calories and need to be limited so you do not eat more calories than your body needs. Remember, if you eat sweets and snacks, eat small amounts.

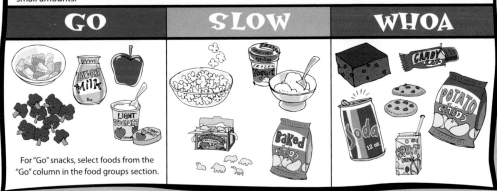

GO	SLOW	WHOA
For "Go" snacks, select foods from the "Go" column in the food groups section.		

Combining Food Groups

Foods we eat are usually a mixture of ingredients from the different food groups. A food can turn from a "Go" into a "Whoa" based on the ingredients used. The examples below contain ingredients from the milk products, grains, vegetables and meat groups – some "Go," some "Slow," and some "Whoa." Foods served in restaurants often use "Whoa" ingredients.

Combined Foods	GO	SLOW	WHOA
Pizza	English muffin pizza with low-fat cheese (using ½ English muffin)	Regular or classic veggie pizza: 1 slice from a medium pizza	Deep dish pepperoni pizza: 1 slice from a medium pizza
Pasta	Pasta with tomato sauce and vegetables – 1 cup	Macaroni and cheese – 1 cup	Pasta with sausage – 1 cup

Move More

To keep at a healthy weight, energy in (foods you eat) must balance with energy out (how much you move). Try to get 60 minutes of physical activity every day. Move more, take the stairs, play ball, bike, swim, walk, and find active games you enjoy. Have fun!

For more information, visit the *We Can!*™ Web site at **http://wecan.nhlbi.nih.gov**. *We Can!* is a national education program promoting healthy weight for children from the National Institutes of Health.

appendix C

a cooking terms guide

You may be new to cooking or have some experience putting snacks and dishes together. No matter how well you know your way around a kitchen, these definitions and photos of common cooking terms can help refresh your memory or teach you a new skill.

This food preparation glossary is also available online for easy browsing at http://hp2010.nhlbihin.net/healthyeating/glos.aspx.

cooking terms

sauté, pan fry, or stir fry

To cook food quickly (for just a few minutes), in a small amount of fat (oil, butter, etc.), in a sauté pan or wok over direct heat. Foods that are commonly sautéed include meats, poultry, and vegetables.

boil

To heat a liquid until bubbles break the surface (212 °F at sea level, lower at altitude). Boiling is a common way to cook foods such as pasta, sauces, and vegetables.

simmer

To cook food gently in liquid at a temperature that is just below the boiling point so that tiny bubbles just begin to break the surface. Foods are typically brought to boil over high heat, and then the heat is reduced to simmer with a lid on the pan/pot to finish the cooking. Foods that are commonly simmered are sauces, rice and some other grains, and dried beans.

brown

To cook for a short period of time over high heat at the beginning or end of cooking, often to enhance flavor and texture, and create a nice cooked look. Browning is usually done on the stovetop, but also may be achieved in a broiler. Foods that are typically browned include meats, casseroles, and anything that needs quick melting and crisping on top.

bake

To cook food in an oven, thereby surrounding it with dry heat. To ensure an accurate cooking temperature, it can be helpful to use an oven thermometer. Many ovens bake either hotter or cooler than their gauges read. Foods that are commonly baked include seafood, meats, casseroles, vegetables, and baked goods (bread, cakes, pies, etc.).

broil

To cook food directly under or above a very hot heat source (~500 °F). Food can be broiled in an oven, directly under the gas or electric heat source, or on a barbecue grill (known as "char-broiling"), directly over charcoal or gas heat. Foods that are typically broiled include meats, poultry, and seafood.

grill

To cook directly over a heat source on metal racks or rods or on a special grill pan. Meats, poultry, seafood, vegetables, and even some fruits grill beautifully.

cutting terms

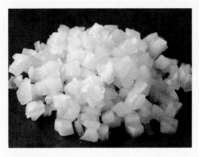

chop

To cut food with a knife or food processor into fine, medium, or coarse, irregular pieces.

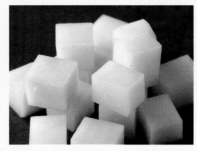

cube

To cut food into uniform pieces, usually ½ inch on all sides.

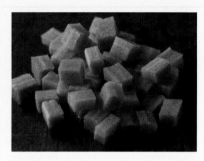

dice

To cut food into smaller uniform pieces, usually ⅛ to ¼ inch on all sides.

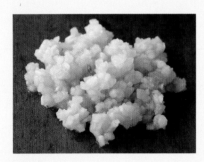

mince

To chop food into tiny, irregular pieces.

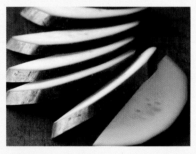

slice

To cut food into flat, usually thin slices from larger pieces.

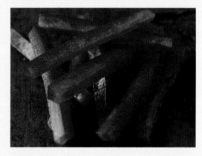

julienne

To cut food into thin slices about ⅛ inch thick and about 2 inches long.

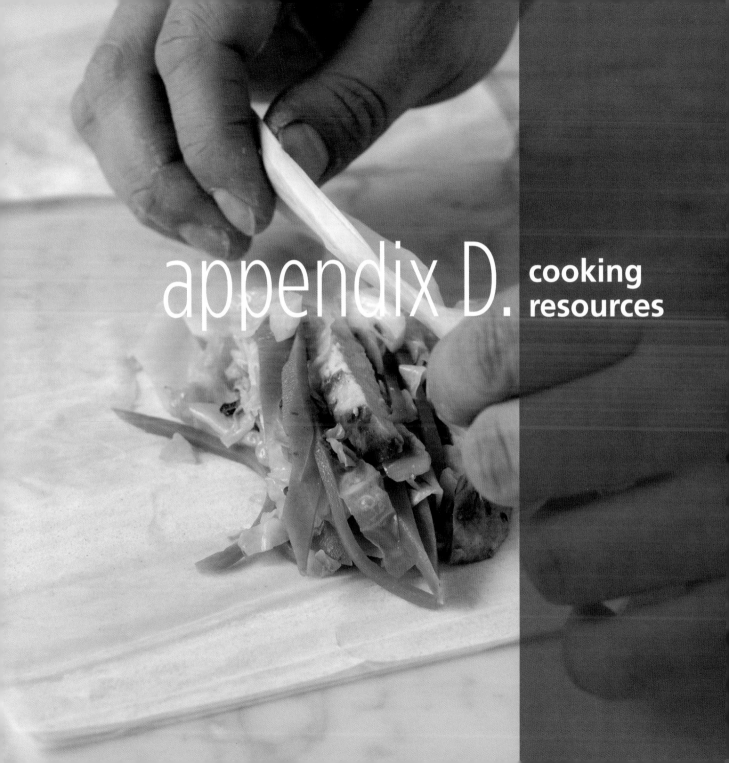

appendix D. cooking resources

guide to common cooking measurements

Teaspoons, tablespoons, and cups are common volume measurements found in recipes. The two most commonly used units of weight measurement for cooking are the ounce and the pound.

Do not confuse "weight" and "volume" measurements: for example, the ounce of *weight* with the *fluid ounce*. They are different measures, and weight is measured on a scale whereas volume is measured using the correct dry or liquid measuring cup. (Measuring spoons, however, can be used for both dry and liquid measurements.)

Below is guidance on some common cooking measurements—and their equivalents—found in the Keep the Beat™ recipes.

Teaspoon–Tablespoon–Cup Measurement Equivalents

3 teaspoons   = 1 tablespoon
12 teaspoons = 4 tablespoons   = ¼ cup
24 teaspoons = 8 tablespoons   = ½ cup
48 teaspoons = 16 tablespoons = 1 cup

Cup–Pint–Quart Measurement Equivalents

1 cup   = 8 fluid ounces
2 cups   = 1 pint
4 cups   = 2 pints = 1 quart
16 cups = 8 pints = 4 quarts = 1 gallon

basic cooking instructions

Several of the Keep the Beat™ recipes use leftover ingredients. Using leftover ingredients (e.g., cooked meat and vegetables) is a great way to save time and reduce your food waste. If you don't have specific ingredients already prepared, you can cook several of these items using the guide below and still enjoy the dish. See the list of recipes in the guide to recipe symbols in appendix A (on page 80).

chicken

Method	Best For	Instructions
Grill (indoor grill pan, electric grill, or outdoor gas or charcoal grill)	All chicken parts	Spray nonstick cooking spray on grill pan or grill racks. Preheat grill pan, or start gas or charcoal grill. Place chicken on grill and cook 12–15 minutes per 4–5 ounces, flipping once halfway through. Chicken should be cooked to a minimum internal temperature of 165 °F.
Broil	All chicken parts	Preheat oven broiler on high temperature, with rack about 3 inches from heat source. Place whole, sliced, or cubed boneless, skinless chicken breast on a baking sheet coated with nonstick cooking spray. Broil for 8–15 minutes, depending on cut and thickness (to a minimum internal temperature of 165 °F).
Sauté or Lightly Stir Fry	Thin strips of boneless, skinless chicken breast	Cut boneless, skinless chicken breast into thin strips. Heat nonstick cooking spray or oil (amount indicated in the recipe) in a large sauté pan over medium heat. Add chicken strips and sauté, stirring often for 5–10 minutes, to a minimum internal temperature of 165 °F.

seafood

Method	Best For	Instructions
Grill	Firmer seafood such as tuna, salmon, halibut, grouper, trout, and shrimp on skewers	Preheat indoor grill pan or outdoor grill. *For fish fillets, steaks, or kabobs:* Grill on medium heat for 7–9 minutes per ½-inch thickness, until flesh is opaque and separates easily with a fork (to a minimum internal temperature of 145 °F). *For shrimp:* Grill 8–11 minutes until shrimp are opaque (to a minimum internal temperature of 145 °F).
Broil	Salmon, tuna	Preheat oven broiler on high temperature with the rack 3 inches from heat source. Cook on high heat for 4–6 minutes per ½-inch thickness, until flesh is opaque and separates easily with a fork (to a minimum internal temperature of 145 °F). If fish is 1 inch or more thick, turn halfway through broiling.
Poach	Salmon, red snapper, cod, halibut, flounder, tilapia, trout	Add 1½ cups water, broth, or wine to a large sauté pan. Bring to a boil. Add fish. Return to boiling; reduce heat and simmer covered for about 4–6 minutes per ½-inch thickness (and to a minimum internal temperature of 145 °F).

vegetables

Method	Best For	Instructions	Cooking Times
Grill (indoor grill pan or outdoor gas or charcoal grill)	Asparagus, carrots, corn on the cob, eggplant, fennel, leeks, onions, potatoes, sweet potatoes, peppers, tomatoes, zucchini, and squash	Rinse, trim, cut up, and precook vegetables as needed in simmering water (or microwave) for specified time. See approximate cooking times (at right) for select vegetables. Use a grill basket or grill indirectly on foil to avoid smaller pieces falling through.	**Carrots** *Precook:* 3–5 minutes *Grill:* 3–5 minutes **Corn on the Cob** *Grill:* 25–30 minutes **Eggplant** *Grill:* 8 minutes **Potatoes** *Grill:* 1–2 hours **Sweet Peppers** *Grill:* 8–10 minutes **Tomatoes** *Grill:* 5 minutes **Zucchini/Squash** *Grill:* 5–6 minutes
Roast	Beets, carrots, onions, potatoes, sweet potatoes, fennel, broccoli, cauliflower, zucchini, butternut or acorn squash, eggplant, red peppers, asparagus, tomatoes	Preheat oven to about 450 °F. Rinse, trim, and cut up vegetables as needed. Place cut vegetables on a baking sheet coated with nonstick cooking spray. Place baking sheet in oven, and roast for suggested time. Use a spatula to turn vegetables when halfway through. See approximate cooking times (at right) for select vegetables.	**Potatoes (white and sweet):** 30 minutes until browned and crispy **Broccoli/Cauliflower:** 20–25 minutes until crisp-tender with slightly browned edges **Acorn Squash:** 45 minutes, cut side down; turn over and cover for another 20–25 minutes until tender **Butternut Squash:** 30 minutes, cut side down; turn over and cover for another 20–25 minutes until tender **Red Peppers:** 10 minutes or until the skin is blackened **Tomatoes:** 25–30 minutes, until tomatoes begin to caramelize

Method	Best For	Instructions	Cooking Times
Sauté or Lightly Stir Fry	Mushrooms, scallions, cabbage, bok choy, garlic, ginger, kale, zucchini, yellow squash, onions, leeks, peppers, broccoli, carrots, spinach, potatoes, eggplant Good for thawed frozen vegetables	Rinse, trim, and cut up vegetables as needed. Heat sauté pan with nonstick cooking spray or amount of oil indicated in the recipe. Place cut up vegetables in the pan. Continually stir vegetables for even cooking and to prevent browning. If vegetables begin to get dry, add a few drops of water to the pan. See approximate cooking times (at right) for select vegetables. *For frozen:* Cook according to recipe instructions.	**1–2 minutes:** mushrooms, scallions, garlic, ginger, spinach, kale, cabbage, bok choy **3–5 minutes:** zucchini, yellow squash, onions, leeks, peppers **6–10 minutes:** broccoli, carrots, potatoes, eggplant
Boil or Steam	Broccoli, asparagus, green beans, carrots, potatoes (white and sweet), spinach, zucchini, yellow squash Good for most frozen vegetables	Rinse, trim, and cut up vegetables as needed. *Boil:* Cook, covered, in a small amount of boiling water until vegetable is crisp-tender. *Steam:* Add ½ cup of water to the bottom of a saucepan. Place cut up vegetables in a steam basket and place basket in saucepan. Steam until vegetables are crisp-tender. See approximate cooking times (at right) for select vegetables. *For frozen:* Cook according to recipe instructions.	**Broccoli:** 8–10 minutes (both boil and steam) **Green Beans:** boil 10–15 minutes; steam 18–22 minutes **Carrots:** boil 7–9 minutes; steam 8–10 minutes **Potatoes (white and sweet):** boil 20–25 minutes for quarters (15 minutes for cubes); or steam about 20 minutes **Spinach:** 3–5 minutes (both boil and steam) **Zucchini/Yellow Squash:** boil 3–5 minutes; steam 4–6 minutes
Microwave	Broccoli, green beans, zucchini, yellow squash, squash (butternut or acorn), carrots, spinach, potatoes Good for most frozen vegetables	Rinse, trim, and cut up vegetables as needed. *For fresh:* Place cut vegetables in a microwave safe dish with 2 tablespoons of water. Cover and cook on high (100 percent power). Pause microwave to stir once at midpoint of cooking. See cooking times (at right) for select vegetables. *For frozen:* Cook according to recipe instructions.	**Broccoli:** 5–8 minutes **Green Beans:** 8–12 minutes **Zucchini/Yellow Squash:** 4–5 minutes **Acorn Squash:** 7–10 minutes **Butternut Squash:** 9–12 minutes **Carrots:** 6–9 minutes **Spinach:** 4–6 minutes **Potatoes (white and sweet):** 8–10 minutes

appendix D

frequently asked questions (FAQs)

planning ahead

Question: How can I plan ahead for recipes that call for precooked chicken or cooked mixed vegetables?

A few of the dishes in *Keep the Beat™ Recipes: Deliciously Healthy Family Meals* call for precooked ingredients. This is a great chance to use leftover ingredients or do some "batch" cooking. Here are two examples:

- The "Fried" Rice and Chicken recipe (page 15) suggests using leftover chicken and sauce from the Hawaiian Huli Huli Chicken recipe (page 13). When cooking this dish, refrigerate or freeze immediately any leftover chicken and sauce or make extra specifically to reuse when you make "Fried" Rice and Chicken.

- The Garden Turkey Meatloaf recipe (page 5) suggests a variety of cooked vegetables, such as mushrooms, zucchini, red peppers, or spinach. You can refrigerate or freeze extra vegetables from previous meals and toss them into the meatloaf, or you can cook vegetables just for this recipe.

The following recipes use cooked chicken or vegetables in the ingredients list, so plan ahead and enjoy them with your family:

- Garden Turkey Meatloaf (page 5)
- Empañapita (page 7)
- Shepherd's Pie (page 8)
- Baked Eggrolls (page 11)
- "Fried" Rice and Chicken (page 15)
- Pasta Primavera (page 29)
- Pita Pizzas (page 35)
- Quinoa-Stuffed Tomatoes (page 58)
- Wiki (Fast) Rice (page 61)

If you don't have leftover ingredients to use in these recipes, see basic cooking instructions on the Keep the Beat™: Deliciously Healthy Eating Web site (http://hin.nhlbi.nih.gov/healthyeating).

food preparation

Question: What are some simple and healthy meal ideas for using various ingredients in my refrigerator and pantry?

Knowing how to choose a few ingredients from your refrigerator, pantry, or freezer and toss them together for a quick and delicious meal in a hurry is a useful skill. Staple ingredients such as pasta, fresh or frozen vegetables, canned beans, chicken breast, frozen shrimp, and lean ground turkey can help you make a meal in minutes. It takes a bit of creativity, but you don't need to be an experienced chef to do it.

See what you have on hand, and try using the basic cooking instructions and meal preparation tips provided in this book and on the Keep the Beat™: Deliciously Healthy Eating Web site (http://hin.nhlbi.nih.gov/healthyeating). Have your kids join you in the kitchen and make it a family challenge—they may surprise you with some great suggestions!

quick and healthy meal suggestions

- Toss whole-wheat pasta with broccoli, garlic, canned no-salt-added tomatoes, and white (cannellini) beans. Season with fresh or dried herbs to taste.

- Make an omelet with an assortment of vegetables (such as mushrooms, red peppers, onions, spinach, etc.), and serve with a side of black beans and a small amount of grated cheddar cheese.

- Grill chicken breasts marinated in balsamic vinegar with olive oil. Serve with a spinach salad and brown rice.

- Brown lean ground turkey and mix with low-sodium tomato sauce over whole-wheat pasta. Serve with a green salad and fruit.

- Sauté frozen shrimp with frozen vegetable stir-fry, minced garlic, ginger, and lite soy sauce. Serve with brown rice or soba (buckwheat noodles).

- Make a salad with tuna (use water-packed tuna and drain it first), sliced cucumber, black olives, crumbled feta cheese, and a small amount of reduced-calorie vinaigrette. Serve with a side of whole-wheat pita bread.

cooking techniques

Question: How do I take the skin off a freshly roasted red pepper?

First—to roast them—place red peppers on a nonstick baking sheet under a broiler for about 10 minutes or until the skin is blackened. Once the pepper is blackened, place it in a plastic bag or bowl wrapped with plastic, and let it rest for 5 minutes. Scrape off the burnt skin and rinse the pepper under cool water. Slice according to recipe instructions.

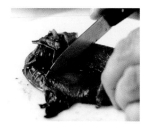

Note: Make and freeze extra roasted peppers to use in Zesty Tomato Soup (page 49), Tangy Salsa (page 51), Super Quick Chunky Tomato Sauce (page 54), and Roasted Red Pepper and Toasted Orzo (page 56).

Question: How do I "fold in" a whipped egg to batter?

"Folding" eggs into batter is a technique used to create extra fluffy cakes and waffles. This technique is used in Oatmeal Pecan Waffles (or Pancakes) (page 39). See pictures at right for how to whip the eggs and "fold" them into the batter.

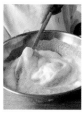 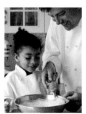

Question: How do I use phyllo dough to wrap eggrolls?

Phyllo dough sheets are very delicate, and it's important to keep the dough moist with a clean damp towel while preparing it. Phyllo dough is used in Baked Eggrolls (page 11). See pictures below for how to keep phyllo dough moist and how to fold the eggroll.

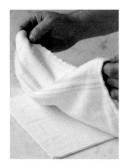 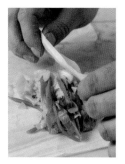 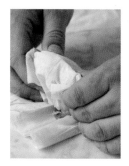

Question: How do I choose and slice an avocado?

Avocados are used in both Tuna and Avocado Cobb Salad (page 37) and Quinoa-Stuffed Tomatoes (page 58). Here are tips on choosing, ripening, and slicing an avocado.

choosing an avocado

The best way to tell whether an avocado is ready for immediate use is to gently squeeze the fruit in the palm of your hand. Ripe, ready-to-eat avocados will be firm yet will yield to gentle pressure.

ripening an avocado

To ripen an avocado, place the fruit in a plain brown paper bag and store at room temperature (65–75 °F) until ready to eat (usually 2–5 days). Adding an apple or banana in the bag speeds up the process, because these fruits give off a gas that helps ripen other fruit.

peeling and slicing an avocado

1. Start with a ripe avocado that is rinsed and dried.

2. Cut it in half lengthwise around the pit. Twist the halves to separate.

3. Tap pit gently with a knife. Remove the pit by sliding the tip of a spoon gently underneath and lifting it out.

4. Peel the avocado by placing the cut side down and carefully removing the skin with a knife or your fingers, starting at the small end. Or simply scoop out the avocado meat with a spoon.

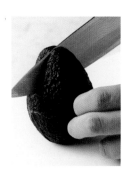 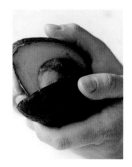 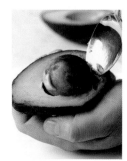 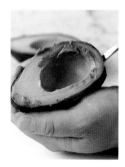

temperature rules for safe cooking

Make sure you cook and keep foods at the correct temperature to ensure food safety. Bacteria can grow in foods between 41 °F and 135 °F. To keep foods out of this danger zone, keep cold foods cold and hot foods hot. Use a clean food thermometer and measure the internal temperature of cooked food to make sure meat, poultry, and egg dishes are cooked to the temperatures listed below. For more information on food safety, please visit **www.isitdoneyet.gov.**

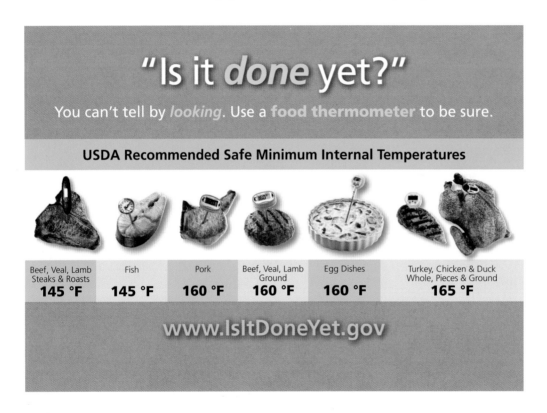

"Is it *done* yet?"

You can't tell by *looking*. Use a **food thermometer** to be sure.

USDA Recommended Safe Minimum Internal Temperatures

Beef, Veal, Lamb Steaks & Roasts	Fish	Pork	Beef, Veal, Lamb Ground	Egg Dishes	Turkey, Chicken & Duck Whole, Pieces & Ground
145 °F	**145 °F**	**160 °F**	**160 °F**	**160 °F**	**165 °F**

www.IsItDoneYet.gov

keeping your kitchen safe

Children may find it fun to help you in the kitchen. To keep it fun, you also need to keep it safe. Following are some tips on how to keep your children safe in the kitchen.

prevent burns

- Teach your children that the stove is hot. Even when it is turned off, children should not play with it.

- Remember to always turn off the stove or oven when done using it.

- Before cooking, roll up sleeves. Loose-fitting clothing can catch on fire. When touching or moving anything hot, wear oven mitts.

- Turn all handles on pots and pans inward so they are not hanging over the edge for little hands to grab.

- Cook hot soups and other foods on the back burners, if possible.

- Food cooked in a microwave can become extremely hot. Wear oven mitts and be careful moving food from the microwave to the counter and taking off the lid.

- Keep hot foods and dishes away from the edge of the countertop so small children can't reach them.

- If clothing catches on fire, immediately do the following: **stop, drop** (to the ground), and **roll** (the flames out).

food safety/sanitation

- Teach children about proper sanitation methods, such as hand washing before, during, and after cooking. Clean countertops and dishes with soap and water after handling raw meats to prevent contamination of foods.

- Immediately clean countertops, cutting boards, knives, and other items that have been in contact with raw meat or eggs.

- Don't put cooked food on a plate or surface that previously had raw meat; wash utensils and brushes immediately after touching raw meat.

- Resist the urge to lick fingers and spoons until the food is completely cooked.

- Cook foods to a safe temperature; test the internal temperature with a food thermometer. (See Temperature Rules for Safe Cooking on page 110.)

other safety tips

- Be careful with kitchen knives. Make sure they're always sharp, and always supervise children using them.

- Keep electrical appliances away from water; unplug them when not in use.

- Put ingredients back after using them to prevent clutter and make cleanup easier.

- Always supervise younger children in the kitchen.

- Work with your older children first to teach them the rules of safe cooking. Then, take a step back and see what they can do!